This book is dedicated to the memory of my dad,
Randall W. Briggs M.D.
and to all the family physicians of his generation
who created our specialty out of the great
tradition of general practice, while continuing
to serve their patients.

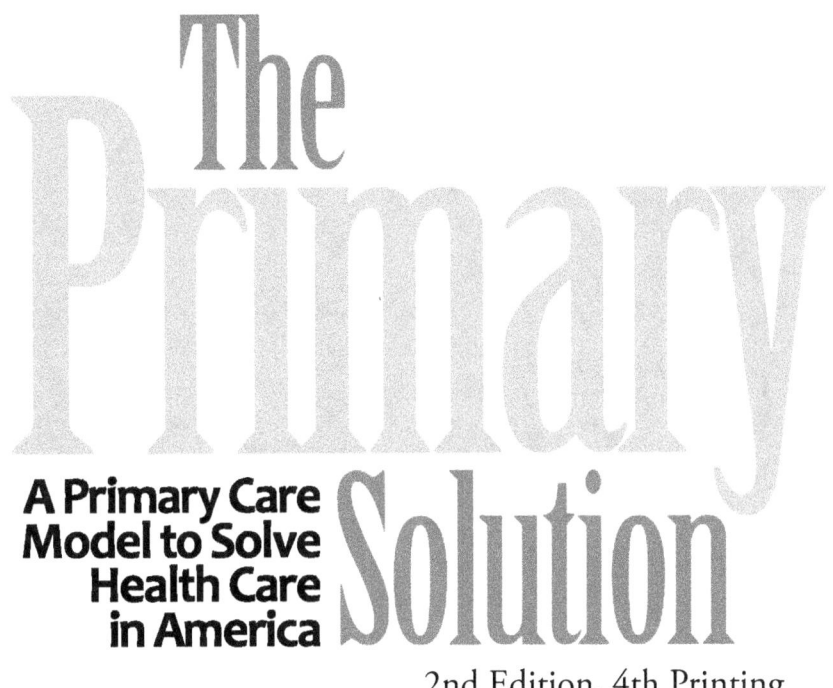

The Primary Solution

A Primary Care Model to Solve Health Care in America

2nd Edition, 4th Printing

By: Philip D. Briggs, MD, MBA

Coauthored by: Philip J. Briggs

The Primary Solution

A Primary Care Model to Solve Health care in America

2nd Edition, 4th Printing

Philip D. Briggs, MD, MBA

Coauthored by: Philip J. Briggs

With Assistance from:
Mike Ries, Lou Bruno, Melissa Proehl, Robert Skinner,
John Chavez, Chris Elliott and Phillip Trujillo

THE PRIMARY SOLUTION

TABLE OF CONTENTS

Acknowledgments   iii

Introduction   v

PART I: HISTORY

Chapter 1: My Story   3

Chapter 2: General Practice to PCMH   9

Chapter 3: The Economy   13

PART II: BUSINESS RESEARCH

The Practice As a Cellphone   19

Value Calculation   20

Healthcare Value Expansion   21

Clinical Effectiveness Index   22

Supply and Demand   23

Diffusion of Innovation   24

Crossing the Chasm   25

S curves   26

Disruptive Innovation   27

DMAIC   28

Porters 5 Forces   29

Porters Generic Strategies   30

Leadership Strategy   31

Hoishin Star   32

Economies of Scale   33

PART III: SOLUTIONS

Chapter 1: Practice Excellence and The Medical Home   37

Chapter 2: Accountable Care Organizations   41

Chapter 3: Lean Six Sigma   45

Chapter 4: Clinical Operations Triangle   49

Chapter 5: Family Practice + Urgent Care   61

Chapter 6: Payer Relations   63

Chapter 7: Health Information Technology   67

Chapter 8: Looking Forward   71

Glossary   75

Bibliography   79

The Primary Solution

Acknowledgements

This book is a compilation of a lifetime in family medicine and the experiences and resources that have been acquired during that time. The list of contributors is too long to include here, but I would like to thank a few people nonetheless.

Certainly my son and coauthor, Philip J Briggs, gets credit for the hard work of crafting the text of this book out of a morass of data and stories that I have given him as raw materials. His style, creativity, and insight from having lived many of the years leading to its publishing will give the reader both clarity and entertainment in a way that I never could.

My senior management and colleagues at Atrinea Health, who are listed as contributors, are greatly appreciated for their help and hard work in creating this new model of delivery of primary care services.

Thanks to my two other sons, Randall and William, and their mother, Susan, for their patience, understanding, and support in what has been a tumultuous but gratifying and rewarding career.

The American Academy of Family Physicians has given me the opportunity not only to serve our specialty, but to reap vast rewards of knowledge and perspective that have given me the unique insight to see the opportunity that is now before our specialty, and be a significant part of the solution to the American health care crisis.

The Primary Solution

INTRODUCTION

So, here is what I intend for us to do:

1. Extend patients' lives and improve their quality of life
2. Solve the nation's primary care physician shortage
3. Double the quality increase that NCQA PCMH recognition yields
4. Cut global health costs by half
5. Double the income of family physicians while enhancing their life style

And here is how I intend for us to do it, and why we will succeed:

1. Extend patients' lives and improve their quality of life

Day by day, a series of events is unfolding that make it clear that we have the tools and technology to substantiate this claim. Probably the best resource for getting a real life view of these events is TEDMED. "The Singularity" described by Ray Kurzweil emphasizes the rapidity with which these phenomena are progressing. Daniel Kraft has the best and quickest summary of the biomedical impact that we are experiencing. It is our intent to be the platform by which these technologies can be brought to everyday people as we franchise and replicate our primary care centers. Sanjay Gupta's *Last Heart Attack in America* thoroughly documents how heart disease, the leading killer, can be virtually eliminated. Cancer, diabetes, obesity, and all the other maladies related to both biology and civilization will soon follow.

2. Solve the nation's primary care physician shortage

The efficiency that is driven by the tools of the Lean subset of Lean Six Sigma is compounded by the addition of a team approach to care in a Patient Centered Medical Home. The time with the physician is distilled to the time and tasks that require a medical license. Eliminating the requirement for documentation by the provider will allow them to put their full focus on their interface with the patient. Adding that to the time spent with the Care Coordinator, Patient Educator, Case Manager, Health Coach, and all the other members of the team will greatly enhance patient satisfaction by creating a much more thorough, unhurried, and humanistic experience. The technological complexity and discipline underlying this experience will be mostly unseen by the patient, but will certainly be appreciated by the more sophisticated of health consumers.

This will allow a physician to easily double their productivity, whether in a volume-based environment or a value-based environment. The experience for the provider should be much lighter and less burdensome, eliminating the hectic, frenetic, overwhelming sense of pressure that often accompanies the treadmill of a busy practice.

Besides extending the capacity of each individual physician, the model will greatly enhance the income and profitability of facilities that are built in underserved areas. As is already the case with many emergency room physicians, primary care physicians may choose to live in an aesthetically more attractive community and travel for shifts in rural communities in which they and their families choose not to live permanently. A robust primary care practice will be able to afford an apartment for such travelers to use in the communities they serve. The centralization of call responsibilities that we have already instituted using a nurse triage system has eliminated that as a concern and burden for the physicians, as has the ubiquitous mandate for the use of hospitalists in any inpatient facility. This change in the scope of practice of family medicine has been the most important one in my career, and although the practice of medicine without inpatient care is arguably more mundane, the benefit it gives to our ability to provide preventive care and to focus on efficient outpatient work is immeasurably valuable.

3. Double the quality increase that NCQA PCMH recognition yields

The daunting requirements of NCQA Medical Home recognition drive an accountability for quality we had never experienced. With a particular emphasis on disease management and preventive services, these requirements, as well as our obligation to track and report them, have imposed a welcome increase in the measurable quality that we provide in our patient care.

I'm convinced that the tools of Lean Six Sigma provide an increase in quality of the same order of magnitude as the PCMH process. Our goal should be that patients will have the same expectation of safety and consistency that commercial airlines deliver. Lean Six Sigma is simply a subset of many other tools of Operations Management, including the Theory of Constraints, Supply Chain Management, Logistics, etc. While these tools have been refined in manufacturing and have made their way into many aspects of service industries, healthcare has been among the last holdout. Hospitals are now embracing these tools and we will bring them to the grassroots in primary care.

4. Cut global health costs by half

The first 25% is already being achieved and documented. The best repository of this data is in the cost outcomes studies being done by the Patient Centered Primary Care Coalition. Many studies are showing results significantly better results. Our first practice data has shown a 35% reduction. Most of this low hanging fruit is the delta gained from reducing ER visits and hospital admissions.

Much more is achievable with preventive care and early detection of disease. Unfortunately, many do not share our enthusiasm for preventive services, most notably the United States Preventive Services Task Force. They have created guidelines that are lengthy, impossibly complex, and are at odds with such august bodies as the American Cancer Society, and many specialty societies. Anyone who lives long enough to see the inconsistency in the scientific literature in a field so complex as human biology can understand why the practice of medicine, and the implementation of that science in the real world, requires wisdom that has been tempered by common sense. Despite their protests of complete objectivity, most of us see their agendas as being heavily influenced by economics and politics.

5. Double the income of family physicians while enhancing their life style

This one's easy… we've already done it. It does require, however, an entrepreneurial attitude. This is often difficult to cultivate in physicians; and particularly hard in altruistically motivated family physicians. Most of the physicians in our current clinics have not been able to fully rise to this level of efficiency. The challenge is to convince them of the benefit that this transition in mind-set is bringing to their patients and to the population in general. Unfortunately, it is an uphill struggle, because the training is so contrary to best business practices and to a profit mind set in general. I have looked for residency programs that both embrace the new model of primary care as well as the need to be efficient and productive, but so far have come up empty handed. That said, I sympathize greatly with the residency directors and faculty that have had to struggle with the changes in healthcare, while adapting to the myriad of different models that residency graduates have at their choosing.

I hope that readers of this book will enjoy the story and take the lessons that we have learned to heart.

PART 1

HISTORY

<hr>

Chapter 1

My Story

The Past:

As the child of a physician, I grew up around healthcare. My earliest memories are of when I was three or four years old; Randall Briggs, my father, was a General Practice resident at the University of Colorado in Denver. We moved from there to Las Cruces, NM where he worked as a school physician at New Mexico State University for a year and continued to substitute for a pediatrician

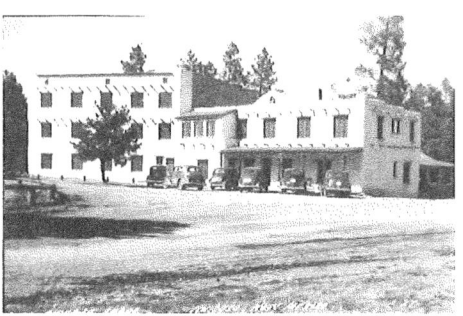

Navajo Lodge: Ruidoso-1958, site of the first New Mexico Board of General Practice meeting.

who had left on a leave of absence for a year. In 1957, due largely to my grandfather's stroke, we moved to Roswell. There my father found a practice owned by Pierre Salmon and bought or took it over; I'm not certain of any terms. It was in downtown Roswell, near the old Masonic lodge. He eventually built a new office close to Eastern NM Medical Center Hospital.

In 1958 at the age of seven, I went with him to the organizational meeting of the New Mexico Academy of General Practice (now Family Practice) at the Navajo Lodge in Ruidoso. I got to know a lot of the physicians there and more about the specialty. This is when my interest in becoming a physician really caught hold.

My father continued practicing in Roswell until he retired. He won the second New Mexico Chapter Family doctor of the year award in 1986.

I left NM for college at Stanford, and then returned to UNM Medical School. I had little contact with the family practice department until clinical rotations in my third year. It was a small clinic tucked away in the back corner of the basement of the Bernalillo County Medical Center.

They built a new Family Practice Building next to the Medical School Library and I applied to their residency program. I wasn't accepted so I completed

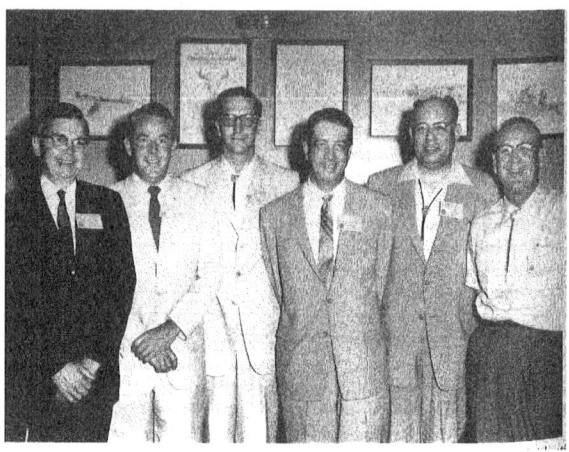

Third from left: my father, Randall Briggs along with the other NMAGP officers.

my first year of residency at the University of Oklahoma Health Sciences Center. When UNM asked me back, I returned to New Mexico and finished my next two years of residency. I then found an opportunity to start a solo practice in Santa Fe. I moved to Santa Fe and established my practice in 1980.

THE POLICY:

Within a couple years I was asked to work with the State Chapter of the American Academy of Family Physicians(AAFP) as a legislative committee chair. I reluctantly accepted the position; it didn't involve a great deal initially but I was rapidly pulled into the succession of officers. I was elected to the VP slot in 1981, then rose to president elect and President from 1984-1985.

During those years I met Harmen Holverson, president of the AAFP, who had come to the annual state chapter meeting in Ruidoso on behalf of the national leadership. I got to know him quickly and he encouraged me to apply for the Commission on Legislation and Governmental Affairs. I did, and was lucky to get that slot much younger than many people trying similar things. I believe Harmen believed I would contribute to the Academy and had a strong hand in the decision.

When I went to the first meeting, the first topic I was to report on was Family Medicine funding under Title 7 of the Public Health Services Act for establishment of family practice departments within medical schools. I, completely naïve to the process and organizational dynamics, reported to the group that I thought we should be against it because I didn't think we should accept money from the government—they quickly straightened me out. My six years on the commission from 1985 to 1991 were great and I got to know a lot about how health policy was made and see it influence the practice of medicine.

I was later elected to the American Academy of Family Physicians (AAFP) from 1994-97, which gave me even more experience in policy and taught me a lot about the general business of family medicine. I then ran for the president elect position and lost. So I decided to try for a spot on the American Medical Association's house of delegates. The delegation consisted about half specialty society representatives and half county medical society representatives. I won the slot and went to my first AMA meeting that was absolutely terrible. They were at 30% membership at that time but I thought I could be part of rebuilding the organization. After a couple more years in that position it became clear to me that the AMA was going nowhere. The organization was just a self-perpetuating one and really didn't, in my opinion, add value to the national debate or to the support of the private practice of medicine.

By then I had become involved in building, operating and eventually selling the Santa Fe Imaging Center. It was an enormous project that I joined into way over my head, but I learned a lot from that experience. I had also started a couple of Independent Practice Associations(IPAs) in Santa Fe. I decided at this point to turn my focus away from policy and focus more immediately on my businesses.

The Clinics:

In 1993, I had expanded from my solo practice from St. Vincent's medical dental building to a larger retail space where I founded Santa Fe Family Health Center(SFFHC) and recruited other physicians and mid-level providers. With a fair amount of difficulty, I brought this practice to break even and eventually paid off all of its debt. From the very beginning we offered both primary and urgent care services.

In 2006, I opened Corazon Family Health, a smaller primary care facility, in Santa Fe. In late 2008, we took over a practice in Rio Rancho, NM to start Albuquerque Family Health. The Urgent Care division also quickly expanded: first with Los Alamos Urgent care; then with NM Medworks occupational medicine in Santa Fe; Valley Firstcare in Espanola, NM; Taos Urgent Care; and most recently Las Vegas Urgent Care in Las Vegas, NM. In late 2010 we opened the first Atrinea Health facility with Atrinea Health Mesa in Mesa, Arizona.

The business debt has been fully paid off for most of the ten years. Our growth has been fairly linear ever since I left solo practice, doubling every 3-4 years with 96,000 patient visits and 12 million dollars in revenue in 2011.

The Business:

The Independent Practice Association has been key to the success of our clinics. We started our first IPA in 1989: Santa Fe Physicians' IPA. I was the founder and the first president, but over the next few years I had resigned from the board and it was gobbled up by Santa Fe Health care, which was a Physician-Hospital Organization that the local hospital created. By that point I had decided that an IPA was the right direction to go in order to leverage power with our payers, but rather than a very large, multi specialty IPA like the first one, we formed a much smaller and more focused primary care IPA with Sangre de Cristo IPA. This organization has served us very well in contracting with insurance companies even though the limitations under the FTC guidelines are significant for the messenger model.

Moving forward collaboration between independent practices will continue to be important with economic forces continuing to push towards consolidation. The Patient-Centered Medical Home platform however, will make a big difference in the ways practices can interface with payers by leveraging much more concrete information with insurance companies for contracting and reimbursement.

Another key development in the success of our businesses has been our business office model. Ever since our expansion to SFFHC, we have had a consolidated business office as separate from our patients' clinical experience as reasonable. Obviously, co-pays and demographics have to be collected and entered at each office, but leaving the clinical site to practicing medicine and delineating the back office tasks has led to a much quieter and less hectic environment in the clinic and the business office.

My wife had traveled with me to many of the national meetings and had heard all the demoralization she heard from colleagues around the country. Because of our success, she encouraged me to consider franchising our model and figuring out a way to replicate the success we had created.

I had consulted with a health attorney in Albuquerque before opening Corazon and they suggested opening another facility and then a couple more every time I went back to them. By then I decided to look into franchising myself and I had gone to the international franchise association website to take a primer on franchising. When I understood it a little better, I contacted an author of one of the articles on franchising, Ken Franklin with Franchise Developments. I was very impressed with Ken and his background of starting over 200 franchises. I flew to Pittsburgh and met with Ken and his wife before committing to the $75,000 franchise fee.

I contacted an IP and franchise law attorney in Nashville who I hired to do due diligence on Franchise Developments before ultimately deciding to go with the firm and committing to the process. The process took two years to create the franchise documents including the franchise disclosure document, the franchise agreement, and the operating manual. We also pulled in another law firm from Austin, TX because I had envisioned the franchise as different from most typical franchises that involve a royalty of between 3 and 6 percent of revenue in exchange for the method and the brand. In our case, the royalty is 17 percent but we provide all of the back office services that franchise law will allow.

The firm in Austin had shared a document they developed that outlined the four ways in which one could create medical practices in more than one state; Those included company owned clinics, management services agreements, controlled physician arrangements(for states with corporate practice of medicine law and a license is necessary to own a practice) and franchising. Franchising was different from the usual management agreement and was a completely new learning curve for our business.

It was about this time that I began the executive MBA program at UNM's Anderson School of Management. During the program I began to seek out references for an industrial engineer. I realized that our method for seeing patients was inconsistent and sporadic and would lend itself well to manufacturing principles. This is when I met Mike Ries, a black belt in Lean Six Sigma and our current Director of Operations. I was in the middle of studying supply chains and operations management so I was able to see these principals in an academic class as well as being directly implemented into our real business.

Initially working with Mike on process change and operations development proved extremely difficult due to resistance from the businesses' status quo. I showed one of my professors Mike's work after 6 or 8 months and his advice was to "Keep pushing, get into more detail, keep going", which we did. We eventually even got into the exam room with the providers, outlining and process mapping every step of the office visit and physical examination. We subsequently used this data and different tools of Lean Six Sigma and DMAIC processing for corporate decision making and continued process development.

Another lesson immediately applicable from my MBA studies came from my first class. The first course was Dr. Sanders' Business Communication, which emphasized the importance of concise communication and targeting the needs of the reader rather than writing to express one's self in business. I had purchased an EMR, Soapware, which had been in place for a year or two by then. I visited with it's creator Randy Oates in Arkansas and trained with the product, but decided we could do something a little better and easier to use. The result started as a audience analysis paper for Sanders in which I used the health record and specifically the EMR to create APSSO, taking the traditional SOAP acronym and rearranging it. I put the assessment and plan at the top because they are the information most important to any physicians looking back at medical records. I added studies before systems as a place for notes on any relevant studies to the office visit, and then put subjective(the review of systems) and objective(the physical examination) at the bottom because their importance is primarily in the visit for diagnostic purposes.

I graduated with my MBA in October 2010 and have continued to find its lessons applicable as my business grows.

CHAPTER 2

FROM GENERAL PRACTICE TO THE PATIENT CENTERED MEDICAL HOME

Though there has always been some degree of specialization amongst doctors, especially between internal medicine and surgery, it was not long ago that generalists in many places were the only physicians available to treat a wide range of medical needs. As late as 1949, nearly 90% of New Mexican Physicians were generalists with only 67 specialists in the entire state. In the early 20th century, medical knowledge was widening to a point where the idea of a comprehensive generalist was becoming impossible. In 1964, the percentage of graduates going into General Practice had fallen to 19%, down from 47% in 1900.

The mind-set nationally changed in February 1969 when family practice became the 20th American Medical Specialty. This reversed 25 years of progress in the postwar medical establishment in which most thought that there would be a number of specialties and a patient would go to a specific physician based on what particular ailment they had. The distinction given to family practice by the American Board of Medical Specialties aligned instead to patients' preferences, who wanted a single physician to guide them through the increasingly complex American medical system.

At the time of its establishment, the American Board of Family Practice sought to train and certify physicians who "would encompass 1) first-contact care; 2) continuous care; 3) comprehensive care; 4) personal care (caritas); 5) family care; and, 6) competency in scientific general medicine." In 1971 The American Academy of General Practice changed it's name to American Academy of Family Physicians to adapt to the nomenclature and the future of the Generalist physician was being reaffirmed.

Education had always been a tenet of the American Academy of General Practitioners and when the ABFP was founded, it quickly followed suit. Unlike other specialties, GPs were not grandfathered into board certified status but could only continue practicing until 1978 without board recertification; every physician would have to pass recertification exams every 7 years. In 1971, New Mexico became the first state to require continued medical education(CME) for its physicians. The state strove to catch all of its senior GPs up for board certification by the 1978 deadline, but when requirements came into effect the state lost a large percentage of its older practitioners.

Though the future of the specialty was secured with the creation of the ABFP, the problem of physician shortages in the field continued. A shortage of doctors in New Mexico and other states' rural areas led to a number of initiatives to regain Family Practice numbers. The rising costs of specialization had the government pushing primary care. There was a national movement to up primary care physicians' payment through the Resource Based Relative Value System (RBRVS). Medical students heard of this and a new force was beginning to spring up in family practice. The national government wanted primary care physicians to be gate keepers to more expensive procedures, qualified decision makers to control patients throughout the health care systems.

I myself had been trying to strengthen ties between the state chapter and UNM's medical school. As a graduate of the residency program, I would buy pizza for groups of medical students to push the family practice cause, and for residents to introduce them to the state chapter. There was a national effort along the same lines and it was a great honor when Bob Graham, Executive VP of the national academy, flew out to talk to the student group. In five years from 1980 to 85, the number of medical students in the state chapter rose from 21 to 90 and the chapter soon met its goal of 100% sign up of UNM residents.

Similar success was being seen nationally as the number of family practice residency programs doubled in ten years and by 1996 family practice was the first specialty to have residency programs in all 50 states with annual graduates reaching 46,000. The elation didn't last very long though. With the pushes for primary care, specialists began to push back. There were physician privilege and procedure credentialing disputes on every scale from the national boards to rural NM hospitals. As specialist grew in number they began to expand into wider areas and family physicians found themselves fighting to keep obstetrical, surgical, and other privileges everywhere.

Interest in family practice also quickly began to decline. While in '92 there were 20 applicants for every residency opening in family practice, the specialty could not fill all of its positions by 1997 and by 2001 could only fill half of the nation's 3000 openings. The government had stopped paying to support family practice, and students immediately caught on. The surge that came with the model of the primary care gatekeepers ended and so reimbursement for family practice providers quickly fell.

The final blow came to family practice as we knew it with the advent of Managed Care Organizations (MCOs). I was a Director with the AAFP at the time and the speed with which HMO's and MCO's grew surprised all of us. Many New Mexico Physicians opted out of dealing with them because they trusted their patients' loyalty, but many patients now having to pay out of pocket left and lots of practices nationwide were decimated. A majority of family physicians had to leave solo practice and find hospital primary care networks or other employed positions with a salary legitimized mostly by their referrals. There was a strong organized effort throughout family practice and the fight continued for surgical rights and other privileges.

I and the other doctors who were able to withhold their practices throughout the struggle ended up on top, but we were on top of a revolutionized method of primary care. We had lost our surgical and obstetric rights, the more fun and interesting elements of our previous practices and were rarely, if ever, required to go into the hospital. Those of us who were able to stay profitable in family practice had found a model providing much more mundane outpatient care, focusing on access and prevention. It was a hard transition for many of the doctors who had to go through it.

Despite further encroachment from sub-specialists, hospitalists and mid-level providers, the prevention focused high volume outpatient family practice model continued to find success. Reimbursement for family practice was at levels allowing doctors to practice comfortably, but was still far less than other specialties. This disparity furthered medical students', whose average debt upon graduation rose, disinterest in family practice as a specialty and residency numbers have continued to decline and the shortage of family physicians has grown out of rural areas into a country wide pandemic.

The Academy, facing an ever increasing physician shortage and without hope for reimbursement increases decided to pursue their own solution. The resulting studies concluded in March 2004 with the publication of The Future of Family Medicine(FFM) Project. The project focused on five major problems facing family practice and developed a new practice model to address them. These were;

1. Promoting a broader, more accurate understanding of the specialty among the public
2. Identifying areas of commonality in a specialty whose strength is its wide scope and locally adapted practice types
3. Winning respect for the specialty in academic circles
4. Making family medicine a more attractive career option
5. Addressing the public's perception that family medicine is not solidly grounded in science and technology

This report introduced the idea of the medical home, a term borrowed from pediatric literature of the 1960s, to family practice, and blazed a trail for what the provider-patient relationship would be in the 21st century.

I have to admit that I was initially skeptical upon reading this report. The "Medical Home" title, as well as the idea of delivering a "basket of services" both seemed airy to me. I've clarified their bio-psycho-social model of family practice by putting the bio in huge font the psycho in medium font and social in small font. Between 2004 and 2008, the model developed a lot and was pushed by a lot of the organizations in medicine. I watched with continued skepticism, but by the time 2 of my practices applied for NCQA patient-centered medical home recognition in August 2010, I was cautiously convinced that it was not just the Academy chasing another rainbow. To me, implementing the model made sense because seeing our patients more frequently and giving them better care would not only prepare us for future value based reimbursement initiatives, but also generate revenue in our current volume based reimbursement economy.

Chapter 3

The Economy

| The Far Left | The Far Right |

Assuming stability in the security of medical licensing and the predominance of western style health care, the economy that a government can dictate for health care has a broad but relatively linear range of possibilities.

On the far right side lies completely a free market for medicine, in which a government controls and protects the rights of providers to practice medicine, but does not provide health care for any civilians or control any health care prices in the nation. In this economy health care is a choice that consumers would be free to reject, and health maintenance would be a personal obligation. Private payers and NGO's would support the medical economy and prices would be set by doctors to meet competitive demand. ER's would be free to reject uninsured patients, insurance companies could deny coverage to whomever they wish, and private physicians could charge what they wanted for care delivery, receiving only the patients or insurers' patients that found their care valuable.

On the far left side lies a completely socialized or universal system of care, one in which there is a governmental burden to supply care to its citizens. In this economy, the government would control physicians completely, determining their pay, outlining their methods and setting up clinics and hospitals through policy. In any government controlled health system, providers lose a lot of their professional autonomy as they are forced to see all patients, but gain a lot of security as policy is generally more rigid than free market support.

Mexico's Seguro Social

Mexico's Seguro Social or social security system is an example of a completely socialized health network. The physicians in the system are employees of the government tasked with providing health care to all citizens. To be fair, there are still a lot of private physicians who charge their own rates and provide care to wealthy Mexicans, but the Seguro social system is controlled completely by the government and relies solely on taxpayers for support.

England's National Health Service

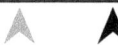

England's National Health service is both the largest and the oldest single payer health care service. A majority of the critical and non critical services rendered by their physicians are free at the point of service, but there are some fee-for-service options allotted to UK citizens. Eye tests, dentistry and prescriptions all require some private payment, but are usually cheaper than services rendered from a private physician.

US Pre 1965

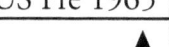

Before Medicare was passed in 1965 the United States health system was largely free market. Providers could see only the patients they wanted and generally could charge what they wanted, barring prices fixed with private payers. Though there were state controlled mental institutions and hospitals for elderly patients, their care was finite and a majority of physicians had little to no interaction with the state systems.

One point worth mentioning is how needy Americans were taken care of in the era before Medicare. The contributions of religious institutions building Catholic, Baptist, Methodist, Jewish etc. hospitals as well as pro-bono work physicians performed as part of their social work were much more prominent before Medicare. In many ways, the system then was kinder to disadvantaged individuals than it is now.

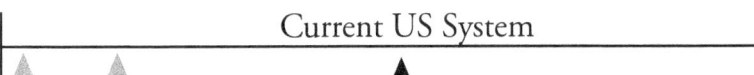

Current US System

The current US health care economy with Medicare is really a moderate system, with a large amount of government subsidy, but a strong emphasis on private practice, insurance and providers. Medicare has changed a lot of how the system works by creating and enforcing payment and clinical standards nationally, even between private insurers and providers. Though they negotiate prices with individual private payers, providers are now generally reimbursed for care based on prices dictated by Medicare's RBRVS. This system is why primary care payments are generally low despite the growing demand and shrinking supply that would traditionally drive prices up. Despite certain demands on employers to supply health care, extended insurance and other benefits are still offered to employees regularly, and a person's obligation to provide for their own health care is present in a majority of successful citizens.

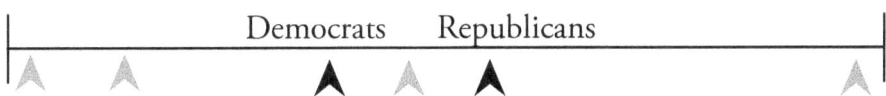

Democrats   Republicans

It is important to realize that though there is a lot of contention over health care nationally, the difference between the systems the democrats and the republicans are fighting for is not extreme. The Democratic Party is not advocating state employed physicians or the obliteration of private payers just as the Republican Party is not trying to dissolve all welfare systems and demand elderly patients pay for all of their insurance needs. Health care is a very important issue to America right now, and though many politicians and supporters are digging in their heels pushing for their system, neither one will mean a complete upheaval of what we have now.

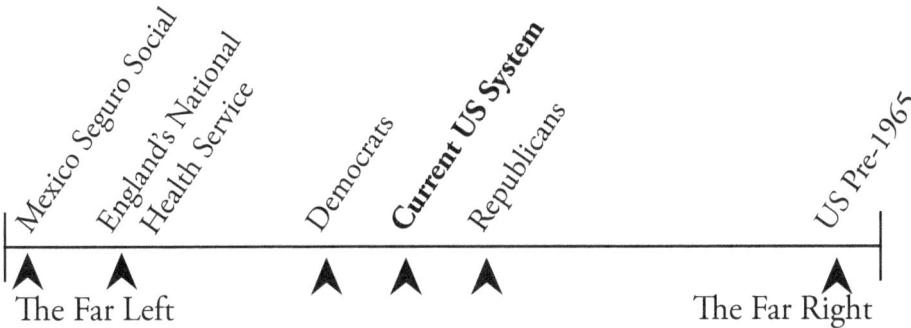

Range for Atrinea Model Practices

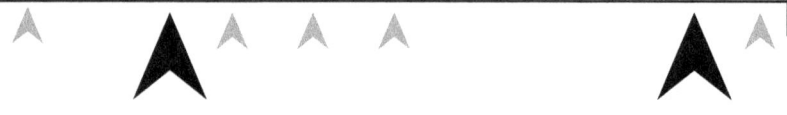

    With this perspective it is important to realize that the Atrinea model of a privately owned Patient Centered Medical Home is an economically support-able entity in any possible outcome in America, especially as we see Primary care to gain ground with reimbursement and importance as a national issue. If the democrats have their way and bring more governmental control into the system, private practices will still function as before, with more federally insured and likely more insured patients in general, and if the republicans have their way and liberate the market, primary care providers will be able to charge more to meet demand and still see a lot of patients insured by employers or themselves.

PART II

BUSINESS RESEARCH

In business school, realizing the new model for Primary Care consisted much more of simple outpatient procedures and routine preventive exams, I realized the consistency of these operations opened themselves to the same methods and principles that have made manufacturing such an efficient and consistent field. As I mentioned earlier, I began this process looking for an industrial engineer to help solve the inconsistent and sporadic way in which providers saw patients. As I continued in these classes, and as the medical home model caught on, my intuition was reaffirmed. I focused a lot of my studies on Management of Technology and took classes afterward toward a concentration in it.

Somewhat rhetorically, I realized and began to say that a Medical Home clinic was a cell phone. A modern cell phone is fascinatingly complex. Today with the advent of the smart phone, designing a cell phone involves a vast array of work from artists to engineers to programmers. Many people see this comparison as facetious or disrespectful to the sovereignty of physicians, but as a physician and a businessman I've found that this approach to management is the most successful way to ensure quality of care while maintaining volume in a hurting industry.

Approaching the clinic as a single piece of technology does initially ring of blasphemy given the respect family physicians are given and due in modern society, but I must emphasize how this approach focuses everything on patients and their health, the actual center of any health care system. In a world with varying qualities of physicians and a movement from intuitive medicine into precision care, modeling a practice to deliver that care effectively ensures much more to the patient than simply elevating physicians does. Every managerial or operational approach that we've taken to practice transformation starts with a simple metric.

$$VALUE = \frac{QUALITY}{COST}$$

This is a common equation for determining value. By determining the quality of a product and measuring the cost, and simply dividing the quality by the cost the value of any good or service can be determined. Insurance companies use this in evaluating our physicians and providing contracts. The government used this(though politics had a large hand) in determining the relative value unit system. We use it to make every business decision; in an economy with relatively low reimbursement for primary care, gathering the most value and quality for our cost is essential to remain profitable while still ensuring the highest possible quality of care to our patients. It's a simple, and intuitive equation, but we make sure to remind ourselves of it with every step we take towards developing our medical homes.

Quality=Patient Satisfaction+Outcomes

$$\text{VALUE}= \frac{\text{Patient Satisfaction+Outcomes}}{\text{Cost}}$$

We've elaborated this simple equation to measure and chart the value of our clinics internally. Here we have determined that quality is equal to the sum of patient satisfaction and outcomes weighed equally. We believe that these two metrics are the main goal of our care. Though some physicians may see outcomes above patient satisfaction, without patient satisfaction and its ability to bring in patients and have them actively involved with our practice our business model would be unsustainable. We have a dual accountability to our patients health, and to them as customers, so we must ensure that not only do we provide meaningful and effective care but also that they are satisfied with our offices and eager to promote our business' growth.

Clinical Effectiveness $=$ (Patient Satisfaction+Outcomes) × Productivity Index

From the value equation we have developed a clinical effectiveness index for determining our individual provider's effectiveness. Though gains share and other movements are beginning to reimburse physicians for the care they receive, we are still operating in a primarily volume based reimbursement system. Because of that, we multiply the value our physicians provide times their productivity to determine this. Seeing more patients is essential for a provider to maximize effectiveness, and creating an environment in which a provider can see as many patients as possible while maintaining a high quality of care is the cornerstone of our operations management.

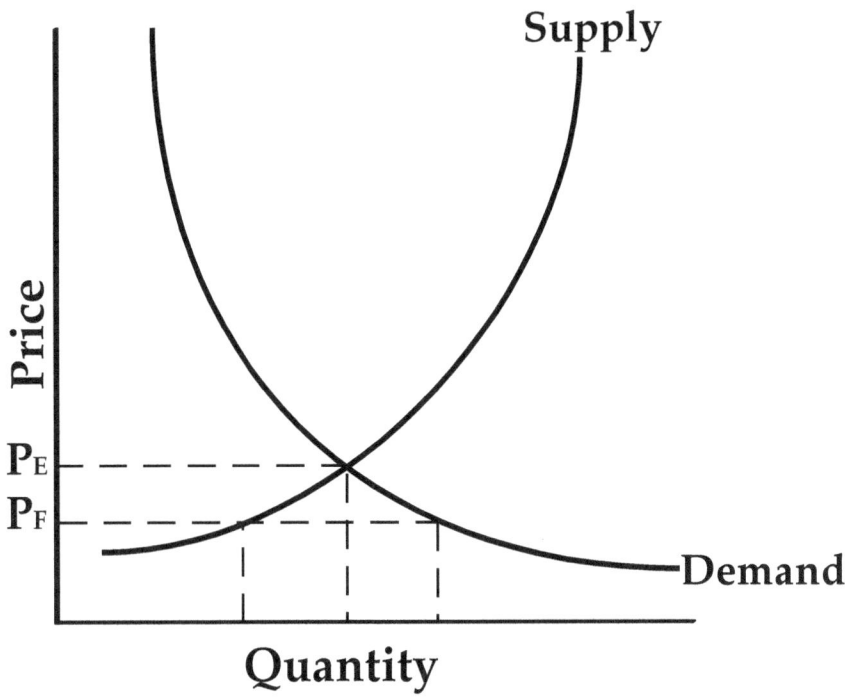

This is a simple supply and demand curve with price on the y axis and quantity on the x, in any free market the price of a commodity will stabilize itself given its supply and demand. This can be seen at Point P$_E$ where supply and demand are equal. A free market will hover around this point. What we see in primary care is a simple phenomenon caused by fixing prices. With medicare and the RBRVS, the reimbursement for primary care services has been fixed below what the market would dictate. The example of this can be seen in point P$_F$. In any economy, fixing prices below equilibrium will cause excess demand, and a shortage of supply and fixing it above equilibrium will cause a surplus of supply. As you can see, the quantity of demand at point P$_F$ is quite a bit above the quantity of supply. In primary care this is extremely noticeable. Residency spots are not being filled, doctors are retiring early or changing field, and in many places it has become difficult to find a doctor accepting new patients or to schedule an appointment.

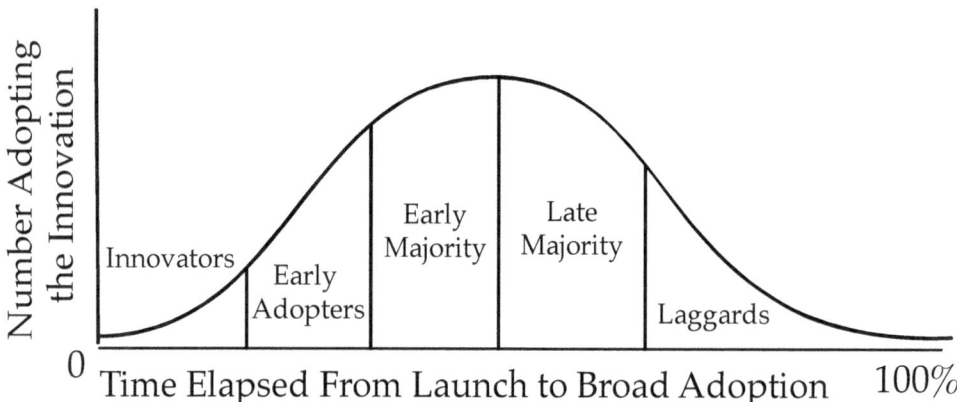

The Patient Centered Medical Home is a model that has existed for years. Very few physicians subscribed to the idea when the idea first came out in the Future of Family Medicine Report in 2004, but as an innovative technology, like smart phones or tablets, we can see it gaining its share of the market in a typical bell curve fashion. Innovators caught on and ran with the idea immediately, often seeming outlandish to their peers, but as we continue to watch the concept evolve and prove its effectiveness, we can see it gain ground and really cement itself as a powerful model for addressing many of the primary care issues in the nation.

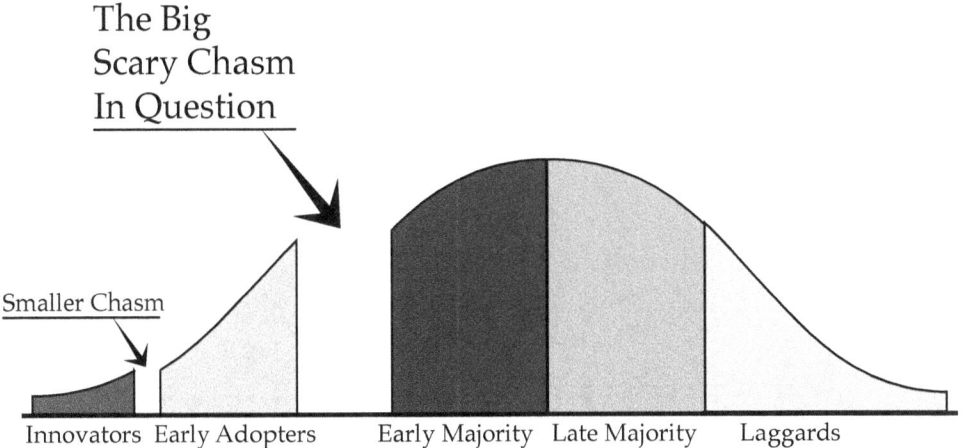

The Big
Scary Chasm
In Question

Smaller Chasm

Innovators   Early Adopters   Early Majority   Late Majority   Laggards

The true test of a technologies is marked on this bell curve as the big scary chasm in question. With every new technology, a rag-tag group of innovators immediately jumps on the idea. A small chasm is passed as a much larger group of early adopters begin to implement the technology. The true test though is when we see a technology confronted with the void between early adopters and the majority of users. You see many technologies fail at this point: Palm Pilots, car phones and beepers all failed to cross the chasm as more useful technologies became cheaper and replaced the need for these innovations. I believe that the PCMH model is just now approaching the big scary chasm, and have faith in its crossing it. Study after study has shown the benefits of this model and we should soon see a wider early majority transforming their practices into PCMHs.

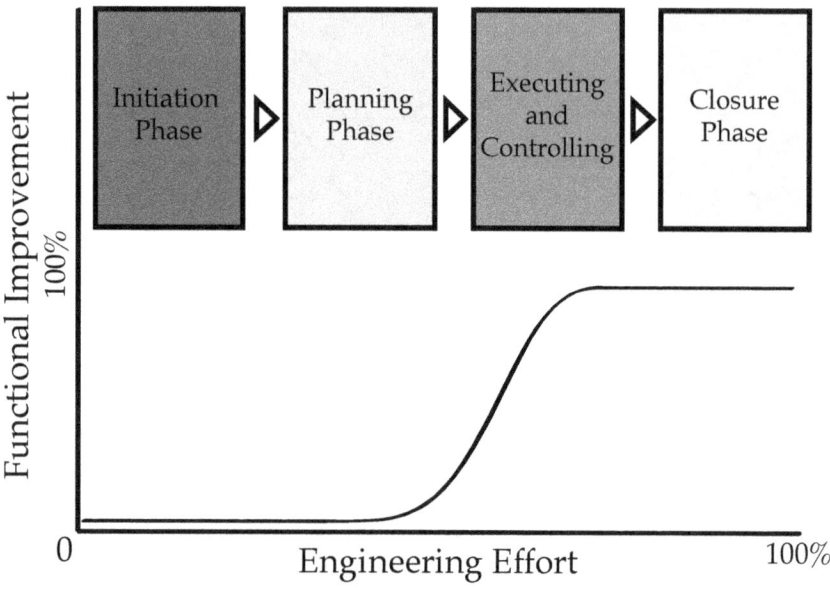

The S curve of effort's payoff has really reared its face with our operations development and practice transformation. Many long, hard and disappointingly fruitless hours were spent developing the standards and procedures for optimizing our clinics before we began to see the benefits really unfold. Unfortunately neither HIT integration, PCMH conversion, nor the leaning of our clinical processes were achievable overnight. Any effective and foundational change we made to our model only came after we spent weeks or months finding our problems, beginning to see ways around them and planning the changes to fit into our clinics. Countless other hours were spent on projects that never reaped benefit. It's a hard road but when the improvements do come it is a welcome sight. We often observe these S curves attached back to back. We have our effort pay off, then find ourselves in another lull, but can push through to even more improvements.

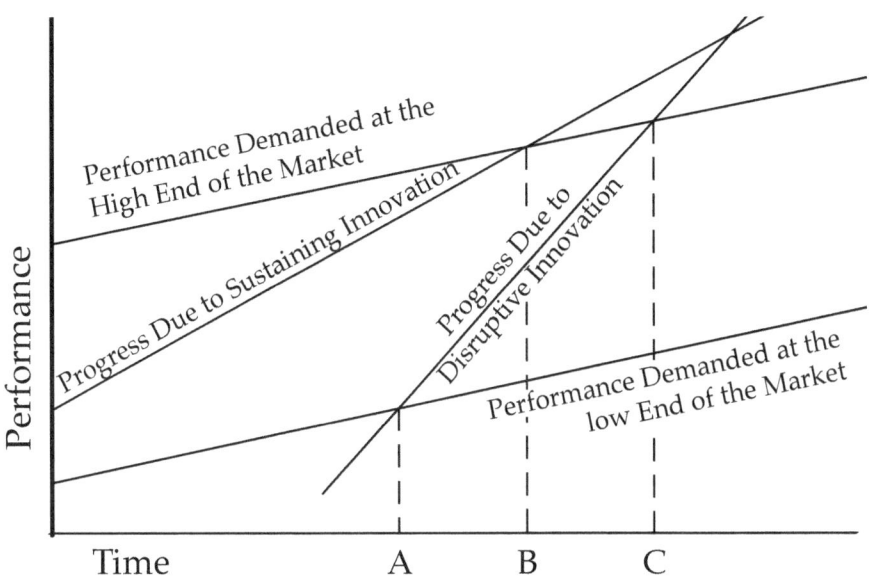

This is a chart outlining Clayton Christensen's idea of disruptive innovation. The two parallel lines demonstrate a market's ability to utilize a technology, the lower representing the least demanding market and the upper being those with the highest demand of the technology. The other lines represent two different manufacturers. The upper line shows the primary innovator, sustainably improving their product using given technology. The lower representing disruptive innovators, who use new technology to create rapid innovation in their products. The points marked are:

a: Point at which Disruptive innovation begins to gain market-share

b: Point when Sustaining Innovation outperforms the possible demands of the product, any innovation beyond this point goes unused.

c: Point when disruptive innovation outperforms the market, eliminating the Sustained market and opening the market for new disruption

Disruptive innovation can be observed in many industries. Netflix and RedBox out-competed old video rental services by utilizing new technologies to cut into the market. Fax machines eliminated much need for couriers and email has outdated the fax.

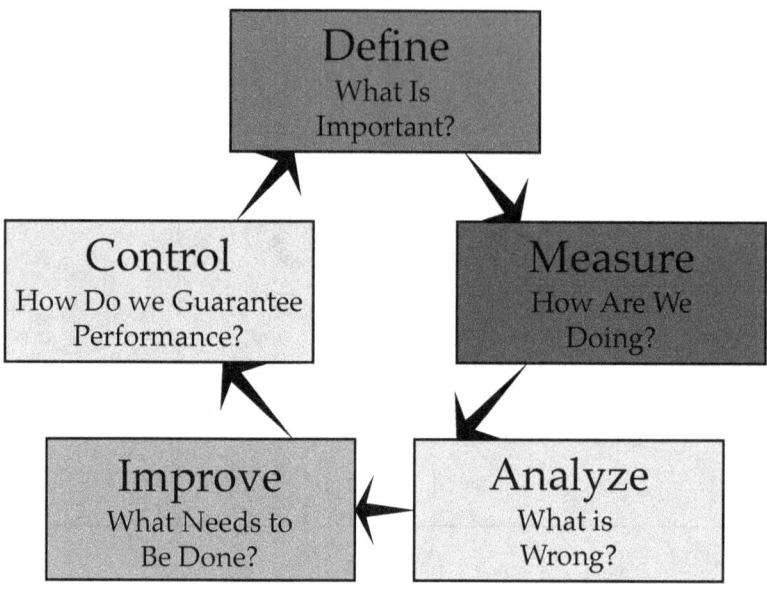

One of the essential six-sigma tools, the DMAIC cycle is a standardized process for continued improvement. All of our business decision-making is filtered through a DMAIC process so that we can take proper steps to improve upon our problems and don't waste time addressing relatively minor issues. All of our operations staff and six sigma project heads lead each project through the cycle to ensure the work they do contributes to improving the problem they've found directly.

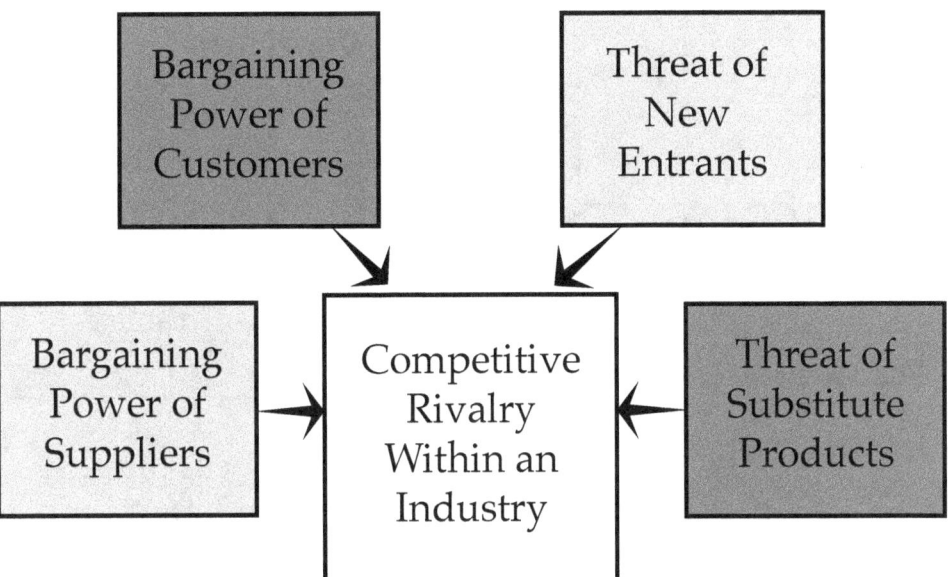

We use Michael E. Porter's five forces model to analyze the PCMH industry. The only competitive rivalry with the primary care industry we find is in small projects like Moore and Wasson's Ideal Medical Practice Model, a model for delivering high quality primary care by seeing only 11 patients a day. Hoping for these levels of productivity to meet the shortages we already find in primary care is idealistic and outrageous. The bargaining power of suppliers is pretty simply the cost of medical equipment and utilities, all of which are quite low for a primary care practice. The bargaining power of customers can come from patients, payers and employers; all of whom are finding little room to bargain against the low prices already paid for primary care and are instead beginning to pay more for proven quality and promptness of care. The threat of new entrants will not be a problem for a while specialty wide as we continue to see older doctors retire and medical school graduates opt for higher paying specialties. But, some physicians are feeling these effects as retail clinics and other lighter options of primary care reach into their areas.. The threat of substitute products is weak but exists in alternative care practices such as chiropractic care, nepropathy, and acupuncture. Altogether, the PCMH model for care finds itself in a ripe environment to continue to grow, and the threats of these five forces seem small compared to the need for primary care in America.

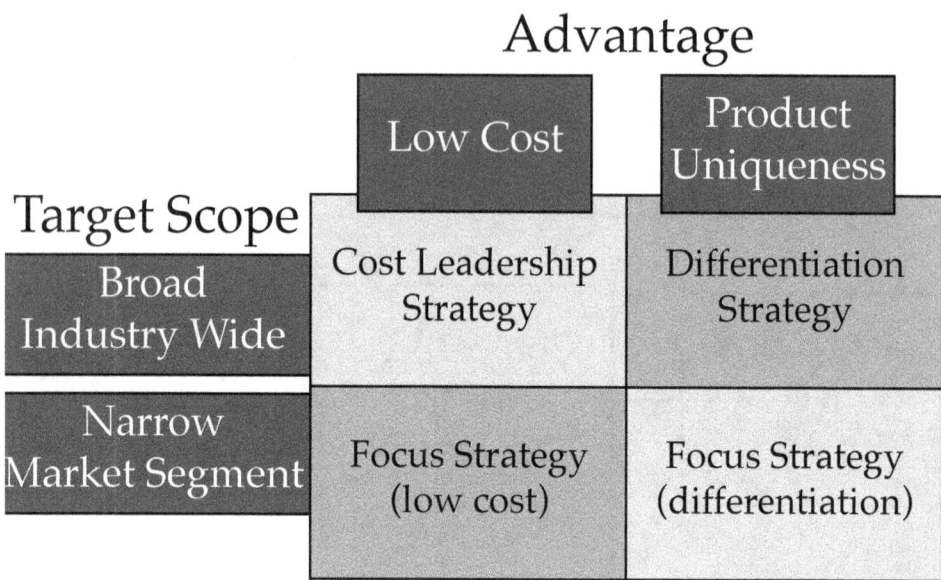

Micheal Porter outlined a number of strategies that companies can use to develop competitive advantage in markets. Above are outlined all of Porter's "Generic Strategies". The strategy that we believe is best to expand PCMH adoption is the Cost Leadership Strategy. PCMH programs are continuing to prove their efficacy at lowering global healthcare costs and will be able to do it as widely as they spread. This strategy for growth will take advantage of the cost saving to payers, employers and patients in order to leverage additional payments and secure their businesses profit.

Learning: Innovative addition of corporate and employees learning and self development, and giving them time on the job for such skill building

Entrepreneurial: Visionary and intuitive elements can be brought to bear in the creative process involving our patients in the process of clinical transformation and accountability in the medical home

Configuration: Most able to re-invent the firm's abilities to serve patients in a world in which Kondratiev's waves are shortening in their cycles and transformational technological and societal phenomena are the norm rather than the exception: in terms of reflexive leadership-ongoing and continuous reconfiguration of the organization and the relational nature of the organization's function

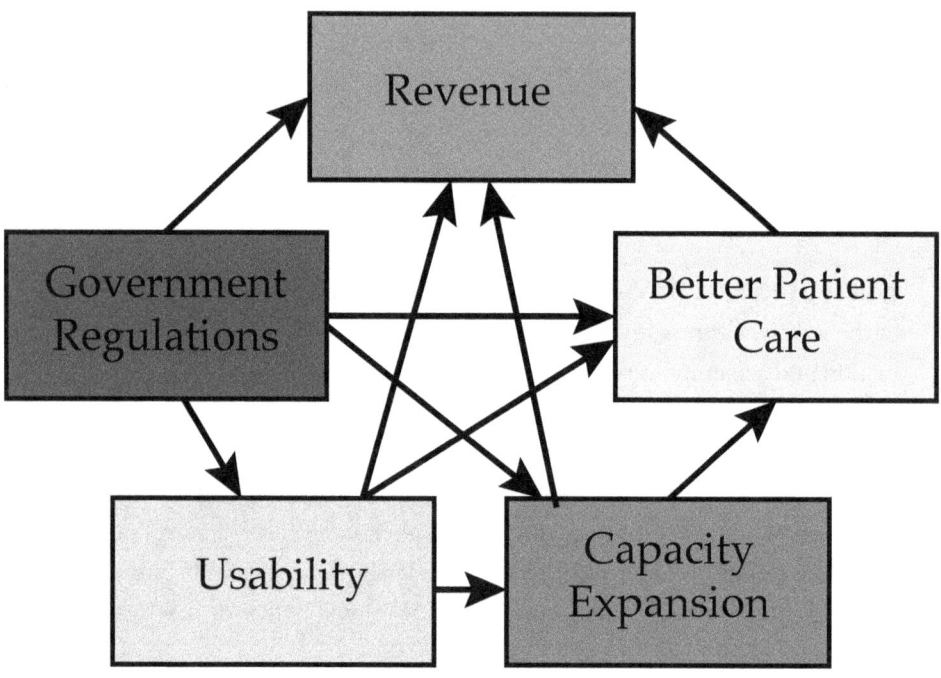

The Hoishin Star shows the forces that exist in a PCMH and how they drive each other. At the top is revenue, all of the forces should coalesce to raise revenue, allowing the business to stay afloat. Second is better patient care, ideally anything affecting a practice should do so to the benefit of the patients health, and we have focussed on enabling this. Third is capacity expansion; in an economy currently short and continually dwindling on family physicians, the ability to serve the population demands physicians seek to expand their network and deliver the same quality of care to as many patients as possible. Next we place usability, our clinics must be approachable and intuitive to patients and our technology must be so in order to drive the higher forces in our practice. Government regulations are the foundation for all of this, and though they are not prime for primary practice, we see a lot of movement towards creating an environment for primary care physicians to reach the higher goals.

Throughout business school, the value of high-level expertise in all aspects of the business became clear. Family practice, a traditionally small-business-minded field, was lacking it. As I saw my business growing, the importance of economies of scale was revealed. With one facility we were able to license an EMR and hire an office manager; with two we were able to develop a light, turn key EMR solution; With four (and our five urgent care facilities) we've created an entire HIT solution for patient registries, tracking, and EMR use, hired an operations manager and created a role for a medical director. With continued expansion, we are able to push a lot of revenue into building a professional umbrella to develop our best practices and fill our clinical needs.

C-level expertise has never really been brought into Primary care; large corporations and hospitals often just eat the lost profits of their primary care programs to gather their referrals for profit. As we continue to grow, these high level tools and personnel will be increasingly within our reach and the medical home model will be refined by these professions. Moving forward I see primary care succumbing more and more to economic pressures, and these C-level officers, possible because of a broad base of practices and franchises, will be able to mold it into a much more sound and profitable business and ensure quality care.

By consolidating our business offices we've been able to develop solutions that cut down staffing in the clinics and relieve our sites from a lot of their previous demands. Our centralized call center has eliminated 82% of the phone calls from our primary care centers, allowing front desk staff to focus on the patients arriving in the office or waiting in the waiting room. It has also allowed us to train a staff specifically for phone calls, making appointments quickly, knowing procedures for emergency calls, routing patients to the best fitting provider and having capacity so that a long and involved phone call does not slow down anything that should be happening inside the clinic.

As we continue to grow, we will be able to draw many of the unrelated task out of the clinic and into our central offices creating a care centered environment for our providers. We will also be able to train our clinical staff to optimize our providers time, as they will be able to take on the clerical and other non-medical responsibilities of the providers. Growing allows us to spread valuable resources widely and consolidate necessary surplus so that each clinic can be fit to deal with any eventuality without being slowed, and can function well in slow periods without seeming overstaffed.

PART III

SOLUTIONS

Chapter 1

Practice Excellence and

the Medical Home

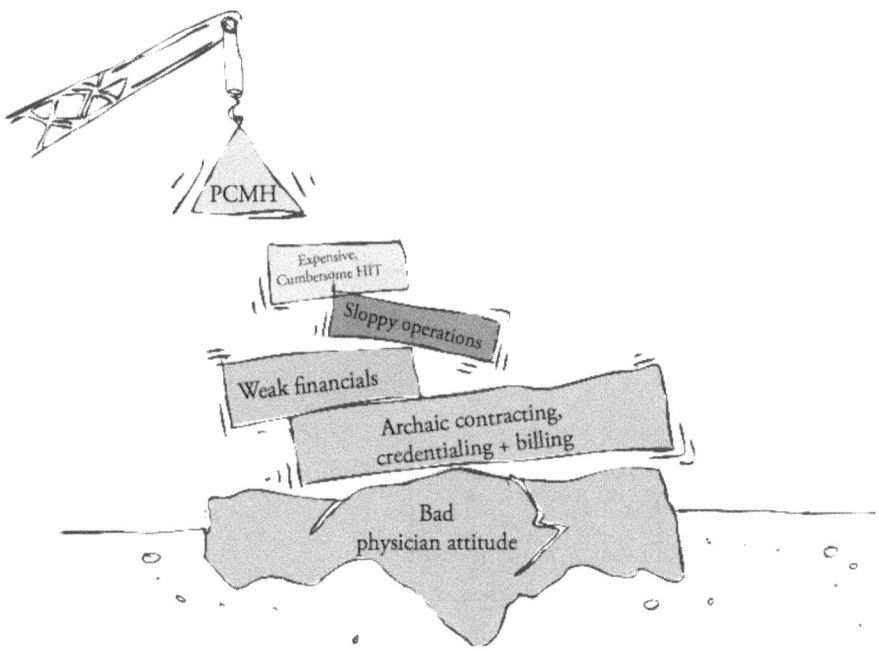

Though the medical home model described by the Future of Family Medicine project is simple, it is important to realize that in an economy where primary care is generally underpaid, building a practice that can meet the demands of a medical home, while remaining economically stable is not cut and dry. Instead of a system of technologies and processes that can be added to any practice, I believe that a medical home can only be successful when built from the ground up. In order to meet the requirements to be a NCQA (or URAC or other) certified medical home and still function smoothly, a practice has to build a framework to support the increasing demands while ensuring quality of care by every other measure.

Providers are the cornerstone of any successful practice. Many providers working in high volume primary care practices see their day as hectic, frenetic, stressful, complex and rushed, often interspersed with lulls of little to no medical activity. The medical home team model allows a provider to see as many or more patients while feeling encouraginly busy, brisk, light, simple and supported. In our volume based reimbursement system, and even in any value based system, providers will not only see the most difficult and complex cases, but will have to see patients with what some might consider trivial medical needs. The medical staff in a PCMH is there to move a providers quickly through the simpler cases, while supporting them during complex cases to keep them on track. Providers will deliver the highest quality of health care if they are able to focus on the patients, and free their minds of the tangential bustle of many practices.

The PCMH model allows for gaining ground in dealing with payers, but having a strong and effective business office is key to ensuring this. Strong IPAs for contracting, quick credentialing, and clear and honest billing are essential to pursue more complex symbiotic relationships with payers. Having this background has allowed us to pursue many new ventures with our current payers.

Financial management and operations are key to implementing a medical home in an economy not yet optimized for it. The easiest way to achieve medical home guidelines would be to just up staffing to meet all of the new requirements, but this solution is not sustainable. Through clear management of funds and staff, a medical home is a model that can be implemented and profitable per se, without the progress with payers. This, on top of the increased relationship with payers can bring the profitability of a primary care practice way up allowing for additional high level staff.

Advanced Health Information Technology (HIT) is one of the main drivers of many medical homes. A lot of software, able of performing copious functions, is available to doctors today. A lot of these extraneous functions can really get in the way of providers in terms of hassle and redundancy. Essential in our medical homes process has been the development and implementation of simple, robust software solutions that meet all of the demands of the practice, while maintaining the ease of use necessary for efficient practice.

Altogether, the Patient Centered Medical Home model is a perfect capstone to apply to a well-organized highly effective medical practice, and its implementation is profitable right away, as well as when it begins to gain support from insurance companies and other payers.

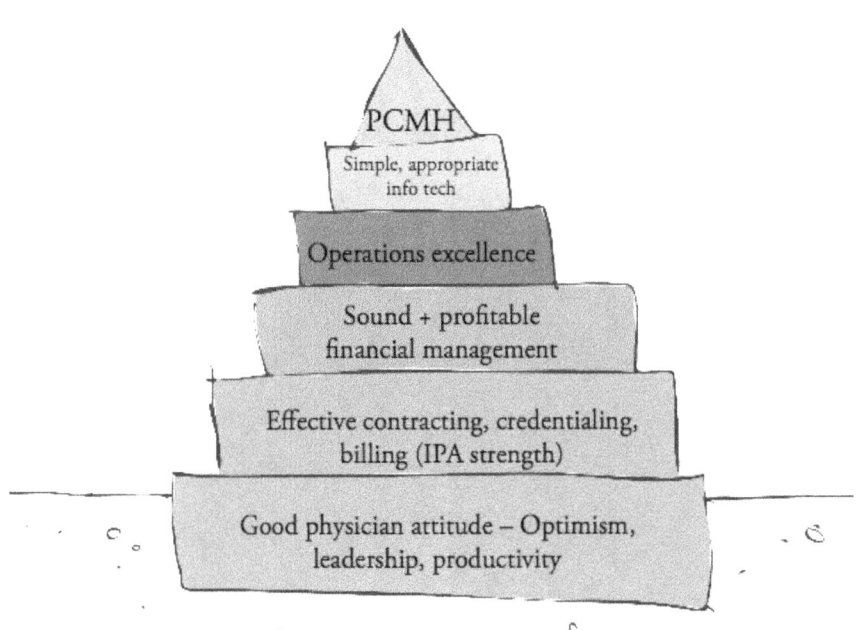

CHAPTER 2

ACCOUNTABLE CARE ORGANIZATIONS
AND THE MEDICAL NEIGHBORHOOD

At the time of this 2nd edition printing of Primary Solution we are engaged with two Accountable Care Organizations (ACO's) - one here in New Mexico and one in Arizona. Both ACO's have been selected and approved by the Centers for Medicare and Medicaid Services (CMS) to participate in the Medicare Shared Savings Program. The timing of our entrance into an ACO, because of our commitment to PCMH, could not be more perfect. There is much ignorance as to what exactly an ACO is, and why its emergence at this time, with so much turmoil in our industry, is important. In this chapter I will describe what we believe is one of the next natural and progressive steps for Family Practices that are forward thinking.

An Accountable Care Organization can be simply described, juxtaposed to a Patient Centered Medical Home, as a Medical Neighborhood. Whereas a single PCMH practice is dedicated to the long term management and coordination of its patients, an ACO is on a larger scale, a range of practices (not necessarily PCMH) that are as well dedicated to long term management and care coordination of their collective populations. The required comprehensive reporting and secure exchange of past and present patient information allows for more precise coordination by seeing a "complete picture" of a patient's health. The benefits to the ACO "neighborhood" - including the patients and their health care provider, are outstanding. The patients enjoy a more engaged and collaborative care management effort beginning with their family doctor. The doctor will be encouraging proactive preventive exams and screenings based upon the patient's age, history and present health. If risks are revealed, the family doctor remains engaged prescribing further screenings and tests as necessary with respective specialists. Depending on the acuity of risk, the patient may be assigned a Care Coordinator who will manage further plans, monitoring, medication compliance and follow up appointments. The family doctor, through shared, HIPAA compliant reporting, continues to assess the patient's path and progress towards health. Through the necessary reporting and sharing of information within the ACO neighborhood, practices will enjoy easier access to their patient's coordinated progress. As well, the remuneration from the shared savings, which I will describe shortly, will help physicians invest back into their practices as needed or planned.

In a broad definition, Wikipedia states: An accountable care organization (ACO) is a healthcare organization characterized by a payment and care delivery model that seeks to tie provider reimbursements to quality metrics and reductions in the total cost of care for an assigned population of patients. A group of coordinated health care providers forms an ACO, which then provides care to a group of patients. -- According to the Centers for Medicare and Medicaid Services (CMS), an ACO is "an organization of health care providers that agrees to be accountable for the quality, cost, and overall care of Medicare beneficiaries who are enrolled in the traditional fee-for-service program who are assigned to it."[1]

ACO's can be made up of primary care practices, a spectrum of supporting specialists, hospitals and insurance companies, but typically have a strong base of Primary Care. Our particular entities happen to be both hospital and insurance plan neutral.

The timing of this movement nationally is optimal for a couple of reasons.

First: The result of the Affordable Care Act, the health care reform law of 2010 set into motion CMS' Medicare Shared Savings Program with the goal of providing better coordinated care for pure Medicare patients. The ACO structure is the means towards that goal, and a financial incentive is built into the program. The shared savings is realized between a benchmark, determined by multiyear historic health care expenses paid by the government (CMS) of a particular ACO's population of Medicare beneficiaries. That benchmark is then compared 12 months later - after a years' worth of focused comprehensive care coordination. The difference between the two measurements - the savings, are split and shared with CMS and the ACO and its providers. This measurement-comparison and shared savings are paid out annually. The savings is a result of significantly lowering health care costs, which is elementary, but absolutely necessary to help save our Health Care system nationally. This incentive based, HIT-driven model sets the pace for the future, targeting the triple aim goal of Better Care, Improved Health and Lower Costs per Capita. Coincidently, our corporate mantra – Access, Prevention and Innovation mirrors nicely with CMS' goals, though ours were codified nearly a decade ago. ACO coordinated care will likely migrate into Commercial Payer populations as the benefits of the current model are publicized and appreciated industry-wide. Obviously, that would yield greater and greater health care cost savings nationally, and subsequently more reimbursement opportunities for participating practices.

Second: As Patient Centered Medical Homes' goals and methods become more known and acknowledged, the standards of traditional primary care will rise. The higher standard will be enjoyed by the patient as well as their insurance company with patient satisfaction rising, health outcomes improving and lowering overall costs. The internal practice modifications and retooling necessary to be recognized as a Patient Centered Medical Home are synergistic with the required reports, coordination and extended care of a participating ACO provider. The two models are harmonious, and I see the ACO as a natural progression of coordinated, like-minded PCMH practices in a region or state.

We are just beginning the initial stages of our two approved ACO's. Within the next 4 months, much infrastructure and organizing lies ahead to support and accommodate the required reporting and sharing of information. Thus, I cannot speak with experience on the actual time investment required moving forward and the inevitable challenges associated with any new initiative. However, I can say with experience, that as with our first recognized PCMH facility, which took several months to achieve, and the time difference with the same task on our fourth and latest PCMH facility recognition, we have learned to successfully complete the requirements in less than a third of the time. The paths to ACO organization and approval are becoming more traveled. And, the number of experienced venture companies willing to partner and fund physician groups like IPA's focused on the goal of successfully launching an ACO are out there and growing as well.

Presently, 250 Accountable Care Organizations around the country have been selected by CMS. That equates to as many as 4 million beneficiaries now covered by an ACO.

CHAPTER 3

LEAN SIX SIGMA

Lean Six Sigma is a concept related to business transformation and improvement that includes a powerful set of tools. The focus of Lean Six Sigma is all about processes; designing, improving, measuring and increasing predictability. Lean Six Sigma is a data driven, and fact based approach for identifying and acting on improvement efforts. It also includes a project management approach that ensures a stepwise progression of efforts with rigorous methodological requirements through the project. Because of these characteristics, Lean Six Sigma delivers strong and sustainable improvement results.

The "Lean" portion of the tools is shortened from Lean Enterprise (or production, manufacturing) and focuses heavily on the customer by targeting tasks that do not create customer value. It is generally focused on removing waste and improving the flow of value added process tasks. Lean improvements can be applied at a variety of levels, from the process level steps to a detailed level of personal activities involved in completing tasks. Despite its origins in the manufacturing sector, Lean improvement efforts are also quite common in service industries.

The "Six Sigma" portion of the tools deal with process performance, developing and maintaining processes that are on target with levels of acceptable variability. High levels of variability lead to process defects, results outside of acceptable limits, which is the improvement focus of Six Sigma. Defects are measured in several ways but often as a percentage or number of results falling outside of the requirements of the process. The name Six Sigma relates to mathematical measurement of sigma (Greek letter representing standard deviation, loosely variability) and that a process performing at "six sigma" has all of the acceptable process output falling within six standard deviations on either side of the mean, or average. Think of a bell curve with a high and low target marked along the curve; 99.9997% of a six sigma bell curve will fit within these targets. Another way to conceptualize this is that only 3.4 defects occur per one million opportunities of a process performing. Unfortunately, the vast majority of processes do not perform at this level, internal processes perform between two and three sigma (around 80% yield) and have to be corrected before delivery to customers who will rarely be willing to pay for outputs that are between 3 and 4 sigma (roughly 96% yield). Improving processes by reducing defects is the focus of Six Sigma improvement efforts.

The common denominator of these technical disciplines is the customer. Lean seeks to maximize results by focusing on steps and activities important to the customer. Six Sigma seeks to ensure process outputs meet requirements, which are customer requirements, with little variation and few defects. It's important to consider "the" customer is actually many people. Customer is used as a generic term for consumers, employees, business partners and stakeholders depending on the process and measurement focus. For our practices, the primary focus is on customers as patients, payers, and employers.

Our Lean Six Sigma journey started with defining customer requirements and developing Key Performance Indicators (KPI's). Customer centric KPI's are critical as a starting point for process improvement. KPI's such as Patient Cycle Times, Patient Satisfaction, Appointment Adherence and Provider Time with Patient are examples of measurement that drive improvement action. Targets were set for KPI's and results and variability measured for each. KPI's that are off target or have excessive variability are the focus of improvement efforts.

Cultural changes have also been important. A simultaneous bottom up and top down approach is underway, with executive awareness and involvement in project selection and progress reviews. Managers are leading improvement projects as part of a Lean Six Sigma Certification program, and staff learns the fundamentals of the process by participating on improvement teams. Ultimately, all employees will be trained either through experience or structured learning programs.

The foundation for improvement efforts is a concept known as process maturity. Processes are the series of tasks required to complete an output of work. Processes are joined; the end of one becomes the beginning of another. At their most detailed level, they look like operating procedures. Processes describe the business activity in a meaningful level of specificity and need to be systematically understood in order to make informed decisions about improvements. Process maturity is a continuum with a lack of defined processes on one end and optimized (low variability, on target) processes on the other. Our practices are in the middle of this continuum with processes documented in a standardized way, KPI's for key processes and improvement projects prioritized based on process performance.

Our initial efforts have been successful and focused on the areas impacting patients the most. We have increased the amount of time providers are able to spend with patients by 50% and are currently working on reducing the variation associated with the patient exam in hopes of increasing that face to face time even further. Provider-patient interaction is a high value adding process, we have been systematically removing barriers and administrative activities to optimize this important experience. Related to this effort, we added a call center and removed 80% of phone calls previously routed to the clinics so that staff can focus on patients in the clinic and supporting provider needs.

We have also documented and streamlined the steps throughout clinical operations removing redundant and non-value activity. The result has been a level of role and task clarity that has provided more consistency for patients. This has been particularly important in managing details related to the Patient Centered Medical Home protocols. Other work has improved patient wait times, appointment adherence rate, clean claims and collection rates.

Lean Six Sigma is a critical foundation for the success of our practices. The investments in time and development of a supportive culture are allowing us to identify, correct and sustain improvements related to processes and, the experience of our patients.

CHAPTER 4

THE CLINICAL OPERATIONS TRIANGLE

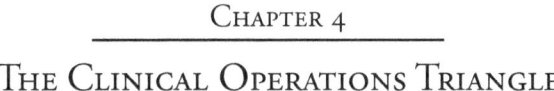

Physician ———————————————— Patient

This relationship is the center of health care. This relationship has evolved with family practice, and has generally been strongest between patients and their family physicians, as they lead patients through their entire medical experience.

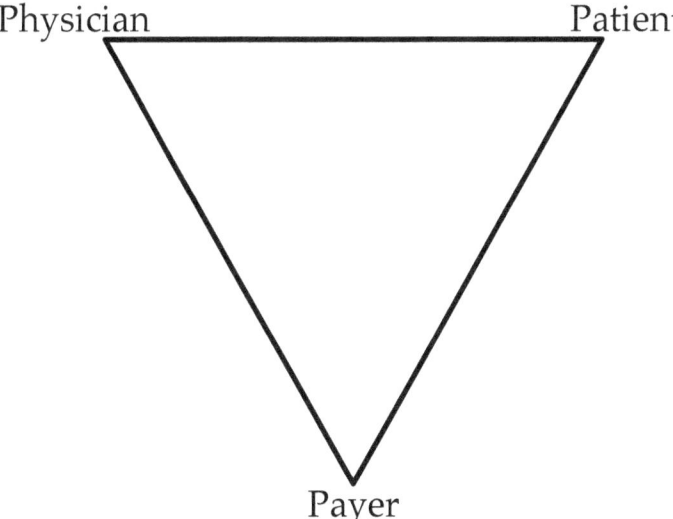

In 1965, with congress's passage of Medicare under title 18 of the SSA, the payer entered into the exam room. Physicians were now dually accountable to patients and payers, including government programs (Medicare, Medicaid), insurance companies, and employers.

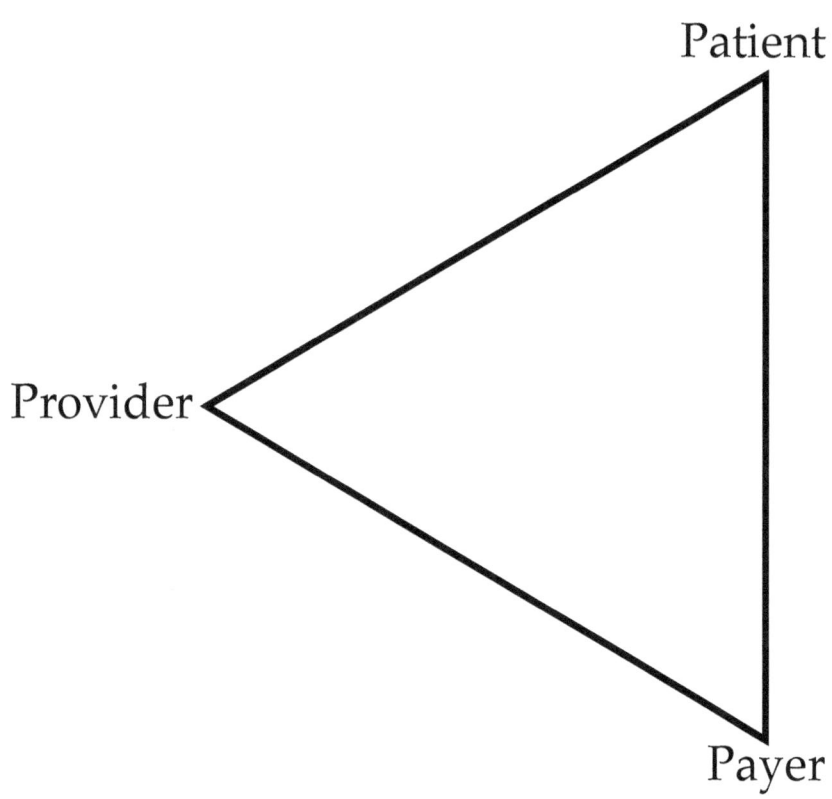

Here we have made a couple of modifications to emphasize our current thinking. First we have rotated the triangle so that the patient is on top while the provider is on a second tier. With the development of the Patient Centered Medical home, putting the patients' needs first is integral in the design of any working system. Physician has also been changed to provider, to reflect the growing importance of mid-level providers (Physician Assistants and Nurse Practitioners) in the delivery of primary care services.

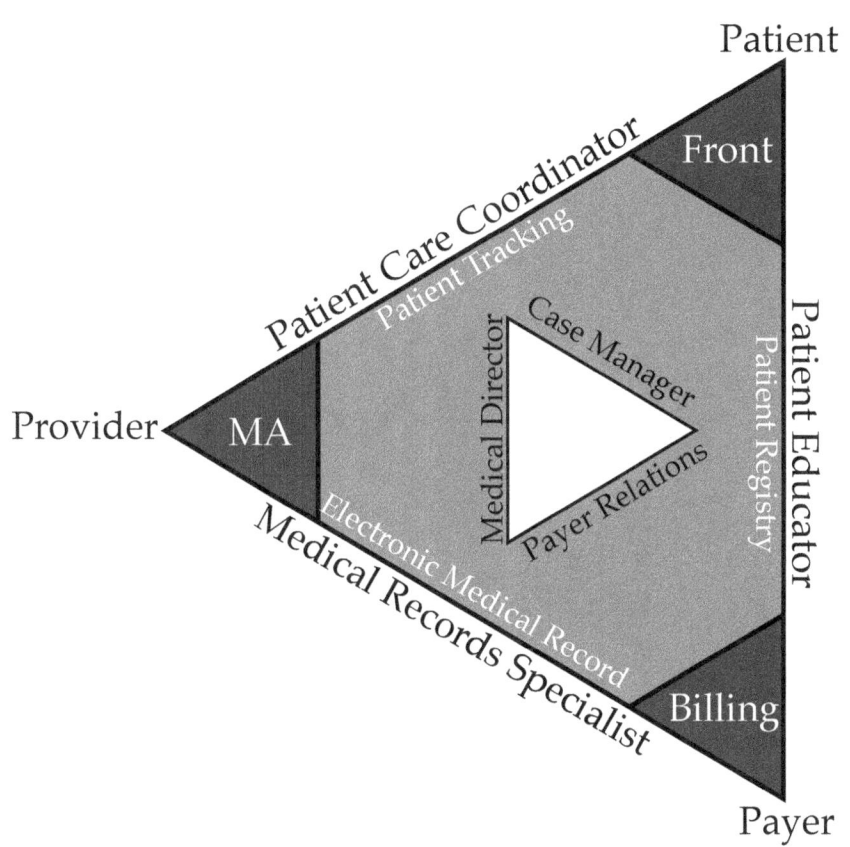

This is the completed Clinical Operations triangle. Filled in are all of the positions that have developed within an Atrinea Model PCMH. Besides Patient Tracking, Patient Registries and the Electronic Medical record they are all personnel designed to ensure the highest quality of care and patient satisfaction out of a primary care practice.

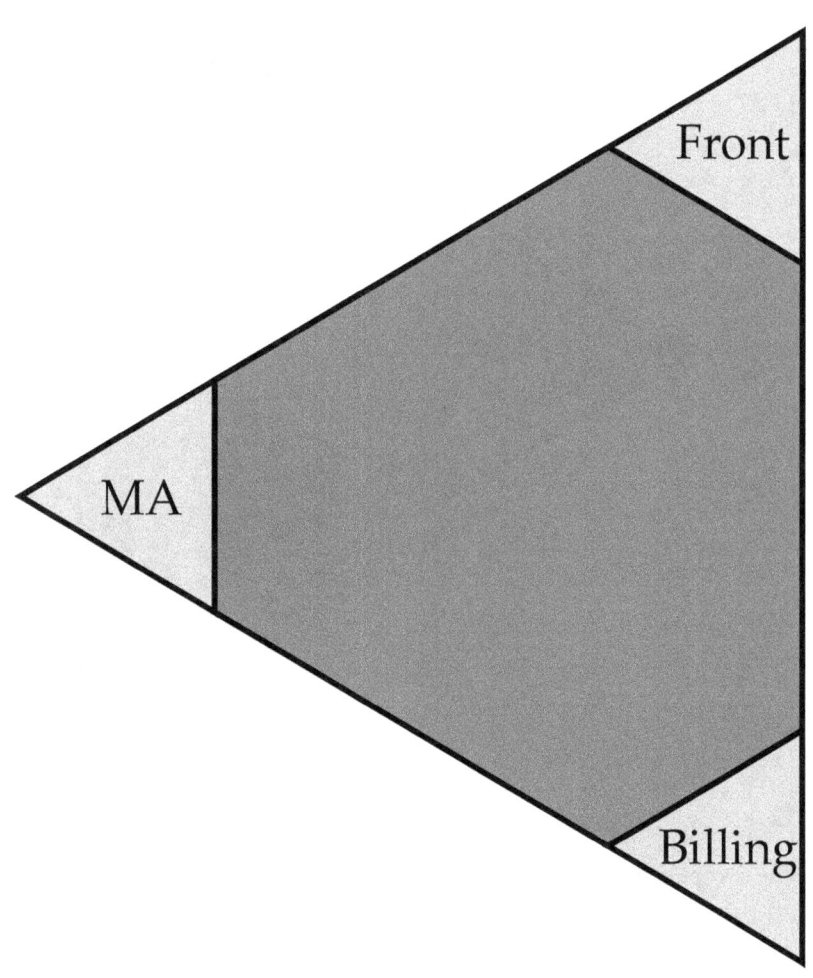

These are essential support staff in any medical environment. They are the staff found in every practice from a solo practice to a multi specialty medical campus.

The front desk staff is essential for guiding patients through a practice. They collect co-pays, demographics and anything else required from patients and communicate to the patient anything necessary before being seen by the medical staff. They are also responsible for check out, in which they enumerate any physicians orders to the patient, verify the status of pending labs and prescriptions and guarantee all of the patient's needs have been accounted for.

MAs are the key support staff for the provider. In the current, and really any, economy for family practice it is essential that providers practice at the top of their license, doing only the tasks that require a providers doing. Doing only these things will allow a provider to have a much more efficient day, seeing more patients, focusing more on the important decision making with each patient, and ultimately delivering a higher quality of care. The role of the MA is to lead the patient through the rest of the office visit. Completing the review of systems, gathering vitals, administering in office tests, and giving vaccinations are only some of the MAs major duties.

Billing staff is essential to any practice that deals with payers, be they governmental, private insurers or employers. With the information gathered from the patient by the front desk and the medical record completed by the MA and provider, they code the visit and bill the respective payer.

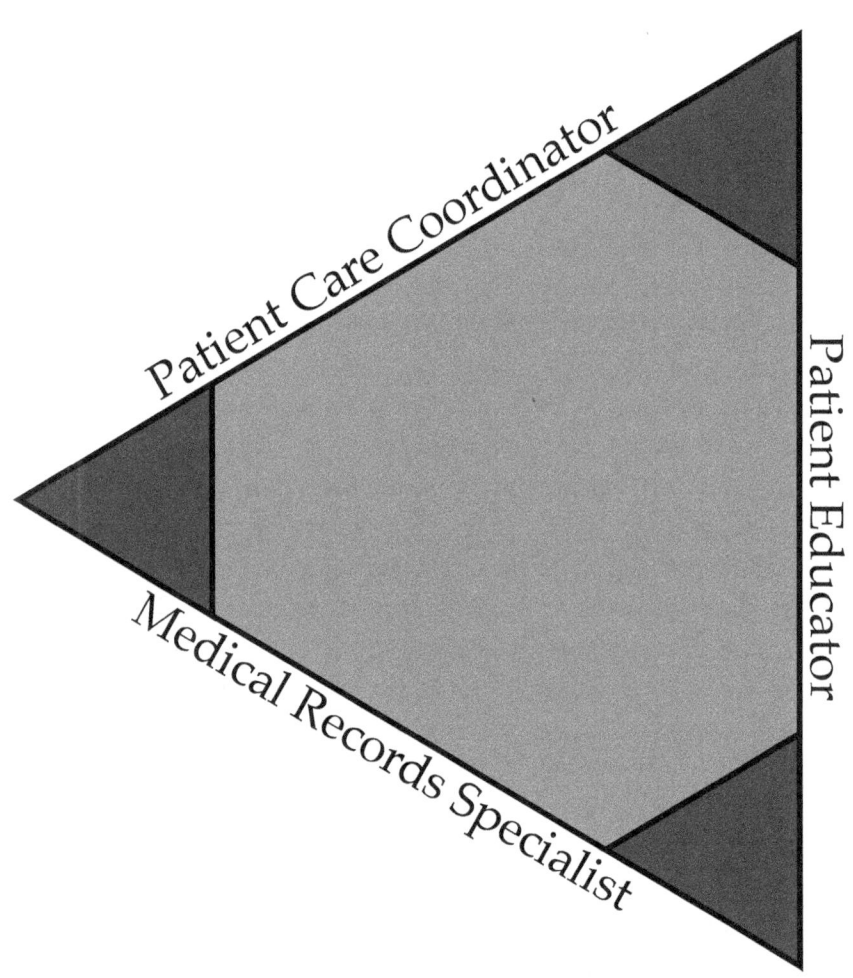

Part III: The Clinical Operations Triangle

The Patient Care Coordinator(PCC) is a position developed for larger primary care practices. They are a convenient and effective solution to the gap between a patient and a provider's staff. Their role is to manage the patients' individual experience throughout the clinic, including labs, imaging, referrals, orders by the providers and the patient's visit with the provider. Walking a patient efficiently and comfortably through the entire visit. The medical qualifications required of a PCC are minimal, less than those of an MA. In the Atrinea Model, a PCC will also utilize our patient tracking software technologies, ensuring accurate quality control and optimizing patient satisfaction with the clinic.

Patient Educators(PE) allow for continuous care and health maintenance for patients with common chronic or clinically important disorders (e.g. diabetes, hypertension, dislipidemia and obesity). Their role is growing and will become even more important with a transition into any value based reimbursement systems. A PE is a mid-level provider who will spend extra time dealing with these complex illnesses. Numerous studies have shown the total cost reduction of patients active in their own disease management. The patient education atmosphere will allow for more thorough, higher quality material to be communicated to patients while also saving providers a lot of time in explaining conditions during office visits. Patient educators will have access to and maintain the patient registries in order to keep up to date on the managed care of chronically ill patients.

The Medical Records Specialist (MRS) is a position of growing importance in any multi-provider practice. With Electronic Medical Records gaining ground in practices, a problem develops in that every provider has their own level of technical know-how and aptitude with computers. Beyond just the health maintenance importance of a medical record, providers must keep accurate records of office visits for legal reasons and billing purposes. An incomplete medical record can cost a practice a lot by disallowing it from coding a visit at a proper level and thus being paid adequately for the services rendered. The Medical Records Specialist is in charge of ensuring proper records are taken and kept of every patient visit. They develop a strategy for each provider to fill out the record, be it by direct entry, dictation and transcription, copying from a paper template, or some combination of the three. Ensuring accurate record taking can really push revenue from billing thoroughly as well as save a lot of headache from the various legal implications of record keeping.

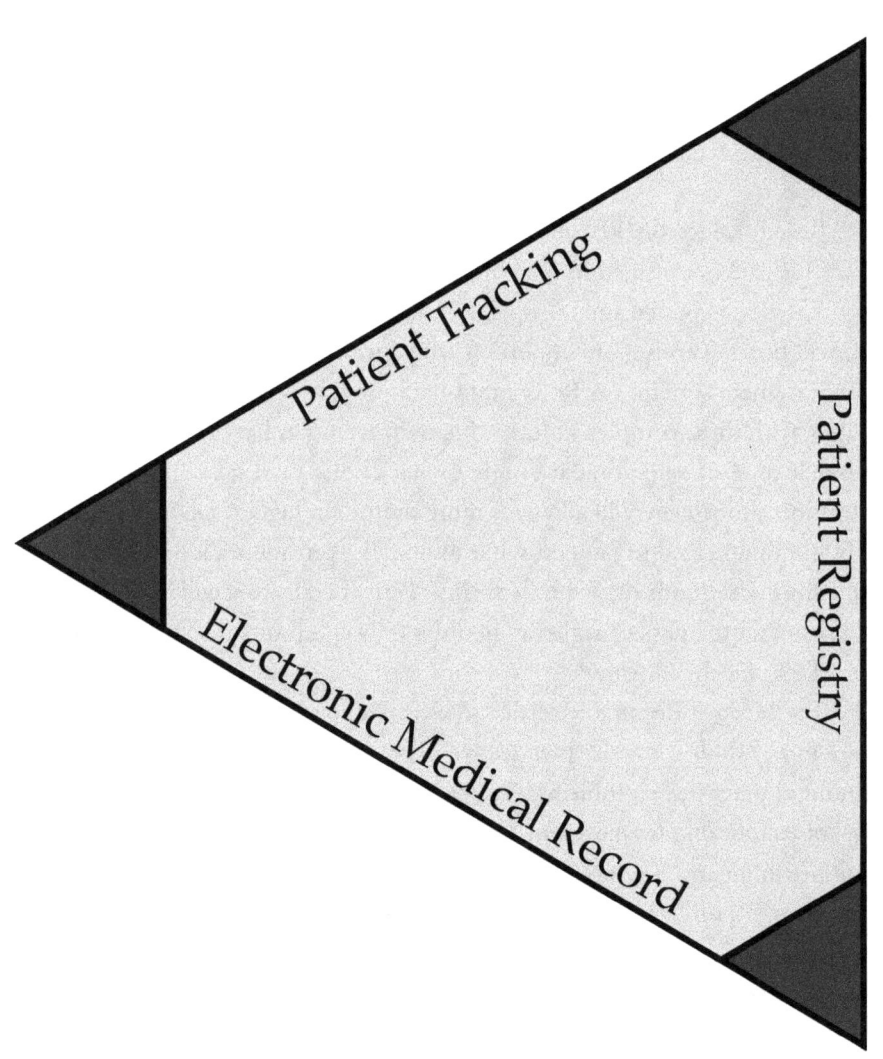

The demands of a primary care facility in HIT are three fold; the patient registry, tracking patients through the clinic and measuring their satisfaction and longitudinal care; the patient registries, tracking health metrics for patients with clinically important conditions for gathering population data, improving health maintenance, and quantifying outcomes; and the Electronic Medical Record, tracking all of the health care delivered and data gathered during an office visit for legal, billing and record keeping purposes.

Patient tracking is essential to ensuring quality of care and patient satisfaction in any corporate health practice. Our patient tracking software solutions track a patient throughout the clinic, measuring the time required to check in, waiting time, time in the exam room(including time with provider separately), and time to check out. It also gathers information from patients upon check out determining satisfaction with all aspects of the experience. Patient tracking also generates lists of patients based on diagnosis and clinical history to identifying those requiring preventive exams, specific often age related tests, and other salient exams. Gathering provider, diagnosis and clinic specific data is essential to quality control because it provides concrete metrics to measure and evaluate effectiveness.

Patient registries are important tools for coordinating care for patients with chronic, clinically important conditions (diabetes, hypertension, dislipidemia and obesity). These conditions are important because; they demand more frequent patient-provider interaction; public health initiatives are gathering population data for continued research; patients with these conditions often cost payers more individually; and an organized, highly controlled plan is often the best way to get positive outcomes. The patient educator requires the data in the patient registry to correctly formulate a plan for the patient to follow. Health insurance companies can use the patient registry data to determine provider and clinic effectiveness, especially in a value-based system. Research groups and not-for-profit companies can compile the data to drive innovation in the treatment method. With these high need, high cost patients an empirical data driven patient registry is extremely valuable to broad progress in the treatment of the disease.

The EMR is the most fundamental HIT solution. All Patient Centered Medical Home models have strict demands of an EMR, and with meaningful use, strict requirements are being put into effect for EMRs. Our EMR, APSSO, will be delved into in a further chapter, but surmise it to say—our EMR is essential to clinical operations and has legal, financial and health outcome implications and benefits.

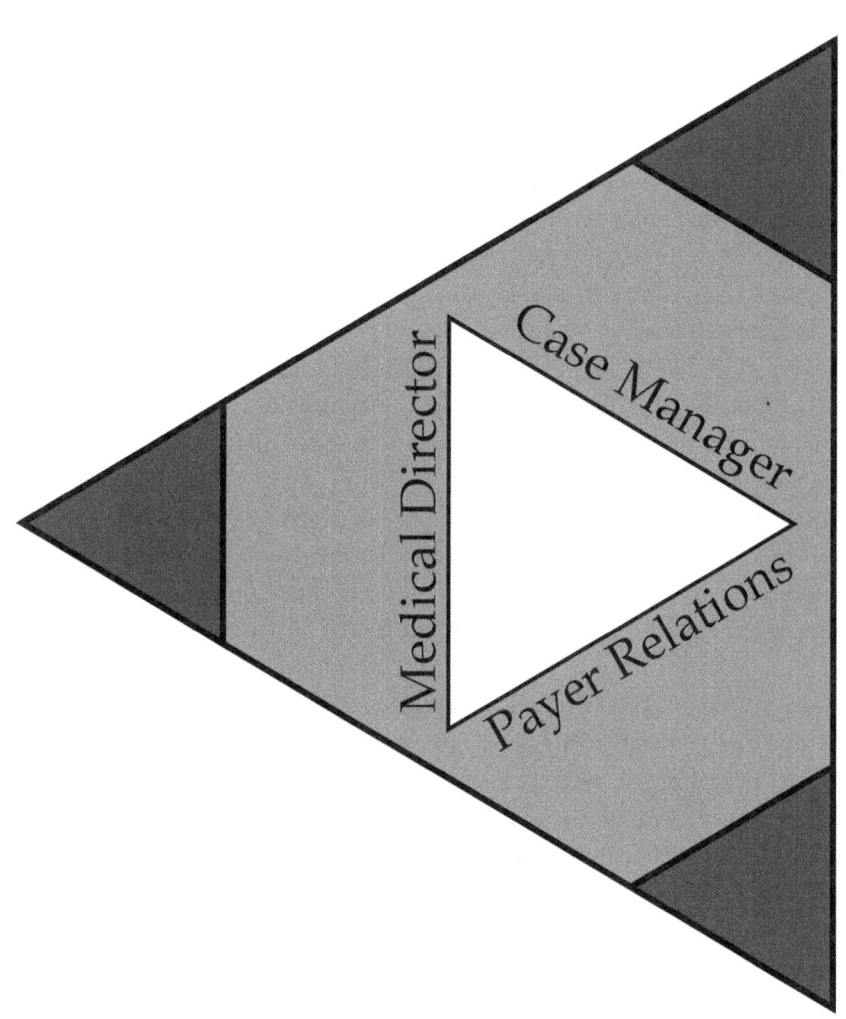

These are the three clinically important roles we have developed that function on the corporate side. They help with strategy for the entire franchise and are important for ensuring quality of care across the practices.

The case managers prime role is to take care of patients with complicated or multiple problems or higher demands for longitudinal care. The case manager is a position that exists in each locality, but not in every practice. In Santa Fe, we have one case manager at our SFFHC location that serves and can be referred patients by all of the practices in the area. With the rest of clinical operations focusing on seeing patients briskly and efficiently, the case manager is the floodgate that disallows a single patient from throwing the entire practice behind schedule. A case manager will generally have less patient volume than other providers, but will also help with other patients when free to. Saving other providers from the headache of these difficult cases allows them to see more patients and focus on their own quality of care while the case manager can take more time to see to the more difficult patients' needs.

Payer relations is a position that began in our IPAs, but is continuing to move into our corporation as we've grown large enough to communicate with payers directly. With the increasing demand for primary care, and the continued shortage of doctors, primary care networks that can prove their value and effectiveness are in a perfect spot for developing stronger contracts with private insurance companies. The data supporting primary care's and medical home's effect on global costs are pouring in, and by emphasizing this while backing it up with your own numbers can benefit tremendously in any negotiations. Contracting and credentialing are the most fundamental tasks of any practice's payer relations, but in the current economy a primary care facility can communicate and benefit a lot more from proactive communications with payers. Payers so far have been very involved with our NCQA PCMH certifications: helping us pay application fees, giving us material to help with application, and sharing information on grants and other incentives available to pilot PCMH programs. Our communication has also helped by allowing quick resolution of any issues arising, including in medical records keeping, patient testing protocols and coding for billing.

The medical director, a position I have filled for Atrinea Health, is the highest level clinically focused position in the organization. Dealing directly with payers, our organization is able to achieve a lot by promising consistent quality in medical records taking and office visit protocol, both of which are important in billing correctly. The medical director is in charge of keeping up to date with current legal and medical information in order to maintain a medically sufficient method of dealing with patients and giving exams so that thorough medical records can be taken and proper information can be used in billing. With the transition from the classic model of a practice into the PCMH some of a provider's autonomy has been sacrificed into the leaning and standardizing of the model. The medical director is in charge of making sure the model ensures patient's care by leaving the most important decision making to providers and guaranteeing staff are completing tasks that they are properly trained and legally allowed to do. Along with the operations officer, a medical director is in charge of designing the entire clinical layout and workflow.

CHAPTER 5

———————————

FAMILY PRACTICE + URGENT CARE

There have been a lot of state supported publicity campaigns in New Mexico and other states for Urgent Care recently, advertising the use of its services to clear busy emergency rooms. Urgent Care as a phenomenon has grown tremendously in the last decade. The reason for this is that it is a simple model for primary physicians to see patient quickly without a lot of the documentation and medical history requirements of a primary care visit. Urgent care services are generally more profitable and demand a lot less infrastructure in terms of EMRs and patient registries.

This all being true, we believe the relationship that a primary care provider, and more recently a medical home can have with its patients is extremely important. The urgent care model accounts well for the acute services that providers can give patients, but primary care providers can see patients for preventive exams, which are consistent and allow for more rigorous patient exams. This relationship allows you to proactively contact patients with reminders of preventive services, age specific tests, and physical exams. We've noticed that in our practices, urgent care visits generally follow national trends, being more or less frequent depending on the economy and the season, while primary care numbers have been consistently growing as the business does, working as a backbone both attracting patients to our urgent care services, but also providing a steady stream of patients in national lulls. The pairing of these services during the day with the urgent care at night has been an extremely effective practice model and has been continuously successful through all of our economic and medical climates.

CHAPTER 6

PAYER RELATIONS

Given the excess demand for family practice physicians versus the limited supply available and the fixed reimbursement provided, leveraging long-term managed care partnerships is a critical success factor for family practice medicine in the changing health care delivery system. With shrinking reimbursement to providers, and payers being faced with an ever increasing competitive environment, cost containment and quality of care are becoming the foundation of most contract payer negotiations and relations.

The key to structuring agreements with payers is to deliver a value proposition aimed at providing improved patient care and satisfaction with an equal sharing of risks and rewards by cultivating a provider/payer environment that creates a mutually beneficial partnership. A provider should build a relationship with the payer that is transparent and collaborative by being flexible and creative in his/her partnering strategies. Contracts with payers should be logical and not cumbersome to implement. And lastly, compensation based on reimbursement models that enhance revenue opportunities in addition to the traditional fee-for-service methodology needs consideration.

Payer contracts that are based solely on fee-for-service reimbursement, or the Medicare RBRVS model do not support the Institute for Healthcare Improvement's Triple Aim for better health out-comes, better care, and lower costs. This is a volume based model that reimburses per patient visit and procedure as opposed to paying for value, quality and cost containment. Value driven reimbursement takes into account the value provided to the patient through patient experience, cost-per-diagnosis or episode of care, and care coordination.

To achieve a reimbursement methodology that is targeted to reward for care quality and patient outcomes, government and commercial payers are entering into value-based payer contracts with family practice providers. Value-based contracting has added a new level of complexity to managed care contracting. It has also added another layer of contract compliance within the provider's scope of services. Billable services are no longer exclusively focused on reimbursing for procedure, CPT codes; but rather, focused on financial incentives for meeting clearly defined quality bench marks. Quality benchmarks include but are not limited to patient satisfaction scores, access, patient outcomes and cost containment. In order to demonstrate the care provided in relationship to these parameters, providers have to create a vehicle for data collection and analysis.

Systems have to be in place to continuously monitor payer satisfaction with provider performance. Although providers need to create an infrastructure to collect and track quality data, overall data tracking and analysis are a collaborative effort among providers and payers. Payers not only have the task in setting the predefined tracking metrics, but they also have the resources and data to compare with the provider data. With this data the payer then establishes best practices with the provider. Ongoing communication between the provider and payer throughout the term of the contract is required to ensure contract compliance is being met, cost savings are realized and providers are reimbursed for the value of care brought to their patients.

How providers are reimbursed for value as opposed to volume and the various reimbursement models are currently being tested. Both private and government sectors are experimenting with a few models as defined below:

BUNDLED PAYMENT: This model encourages care coordination among providers. Part A and Part B providers are reimbursed for their efforts and share a single, fixed-payment for services.

Shared-Savings Models: This model places the family practice physician at the core of care coordination with a focus on preventive care. It is a model being tested with hospital and physician providers forming Accountable Care Organizations. It encourages providers to reduce overall healthcare spending below the level set forth by the payer by rewarding the provider with the shared savings.

PAY-FOR PERFORMANCE: This model pays for the provider meeting specific quality and cost metrics and can be paid based on a per member per month basis in addition to the provider's fee-for-service rate.

CAPITATED: This model is based on a fixed-fee, per member per month fee to manage all health care needs for a given patient population.

Even though different schools of thought exist with regards to what payment models are the best, most would agree that traditional fee-for-service reimbursement methodology is not sustainable in driving change in the healthcare delivery system. Family practice physicians need to prepare their practices to not depend on volume to secure revenue but rather value of care for reimbursement. They must align clinical care management programs to physician care planning to bring value to their patients with an aim at lowering overall healthcare costs.

HOW IT WORKS:

Providers have to consider payers as customers by assessing and meeting their needs. Perceiving the payers as partners may be counter intuitive for many providers. But, by fostering a positive relationship with payers, a provider positions his/herself at an advantage. A payer is more inclined to work toward a mutually beneficial agreement for the provider and payer within a positive payer relationship as opposed to a negative one. When negotiating a contract and rates, a positive payer relationship aids in gathering information so a provider can establish a clear assessment around a managed care strategy and market pricing. In addition, it is important providers establish an understanding as to which payers to build long-standing relationships with, and which ones don't fit within their organizational strategy.

A positive provider reputation is built upon consistency, transparency and responsiveness. Maintaining your payer relationship is equally important to creating a payer relationship. Ongoing payer meetings assist with surveying how things are going. Exchanging information and payer audits creates transparency. Lastly, being responsive with action items to member grievances and or billing issues helps to build payer trust.

To assist with continuous quality improvement efforts, a task committee comprising of clinical, financial and operational team members that meet quarterly is essential. This committee comprises of executive team members from both the payer and provider side. This committee is responsible for determining not only if the provider is meeting the payer's needs but also what the payer can do to meet the needs of the provider. This committee is tasked with addressing ongoing operational or any other issues that can potentially negatively impact the relationship. The quarterly meetings assist with being proactive as opposed to reactive to issues that otherwise might have been an unfortunate surprise to both parties.

The results of viewing the payer as a customer is a long-term provider/payer relationship built around trust and mutual goals. Subsequently, this relationship is a driver in transforming the healthcare delivery system around patient satisfaction, better care and lower costs.

CHAPTER 7

HEALTH INFORMATION TECHNOLOGY

As stated earlier, a well-organized highly effective medical practice needs to include simple and appropriate HIT. Thus, the fundamental tenets for health information technology must include ease of use and transparency. Ease of use is a practical necessity for the provider and the rest of the care team, and transparency is critical in that information technology must be as non-intrusive as possible. In other words, the information technology must enable the individual to perform to the maximum of their profession, while not interfering with the primary goal.

Within the setting of the Patient Centered Medical Home, these tenets are achieved by having the health information technologist carefully examine the requirements of each stakeholder in the Clinical Operations Triangle, first at the individual functional view, and then from a systems perspective. In addition, there must be consideration of the inter-relationship of the people-process-technology triad. For example, what training, staff roles, processes and technology should be brought to bear to enable the provider to practice at the top of her/his license. This approach should also be taken for each of the other roles (i.e. medical assistants, patient care coordinators, etc.). Lastly, the health-care information technologist must ensure the choices interoperate effectively in order to achieve a highly functional, efficient and supportable system.

We are sourcing and selecting the information technologies that enable us to achieve the above stated goals and tenets. While building and managing the information technology system, we are also keeping attuned to the emerging technologies that can enable substantial improvement in the PCMH setting. For example, what if the provider had inexpensive and real-time access to essential information not available today like labs (i.e. "lab in a box"), genomic sequencing, and coronary cross-sectional imaging? Would that not be transformational for the quality and cost of care? What if the patient practice had the technologies that enabled immediate access to up-to-date patient information at the time the patient stepped into the clinic door, so that the staff could immediately place the patient directly into the exam room? Would that not be transformational for patient satisfaction, and clinic efficiency? Therefore, another role of the health information technologist includes the constant research for and review of potential technologies both inside and outside of healthcare.

Our goal of simple and appropriate HIT must also take into consideration business requirements such as profitable growth, PCMH certification, and Accountable Care Organization compliance. In addition, we must meet the requirements for government mandated programs such as the Health Insurance Portability and Accountability Act (HIPAA) and the Patient Protection and Affordable Care Act (PPACA). These initiatives go a long way toward enabling the healthcare system as a whole to provide higher quality patient care. However, we are careful to keep our basic tenets and goals in the forefront as we deal with requirements of the government mandates. For example, HIPAA Privacy and Security requirements have grown stricter, which can encroach upon ease of use and simplicity, so we seek technologies that enable us to achieve both. Another example is Meaningful Use, and the associated monetary incentives. As illustrated in the table below, our focus on efficiency and increasing capacity to enable providers to see more patients per day trumps the Meaningful Use payouts. We totaled the maximum possible payout for meaningful use payments for nine providers, and compared it with the chance of seeing just one more patient per day (at a medium coding level).

	EPs	Year 1	Year 2	Year 3	Year 4	Year 5	Total
Incenti ve Payments	9	$ 191,250	$ 76,500	$ 76,500	$ 76,500	$ 76,500	$ 497,250
One More Pati ent per Day	9	$ 249,480	$ 249,480	$ 249,480	$ 249,480	$ 249,480	$ 1,247,400

As you can see, the meaningful use payments are substantial, and could net us nearly five hundred thousand dollars over four years, but it doesn't come close to the financial benefits of enabling a provider to see more patients. And furthermore, increased patient volume enables us to apply best practice to larger patient population thereby increasing the reach and impact of quality patient care. Therefore, while we are pursuing meaningful-user attestation, that remains secondary to our primary goal of the adoption and use of simple and easy to use technology that supports operational efficiency and clinical capability to see more patients.

CHAPTER 8

LOOKING FORWARD

With specialization and the managed care phenomenon, general practice and family practice have lost a lot of their hospital rights and privileges. The practice has transformed since the beginning of the 20th century into outpatient, prevention focused and minor acute services. I feel like the tide is about to change as certain previously prohibitively expensive tests are going through Christensen's process of disruptive innovation and are becoming cheap enough and valuable enough to be everyday. Tests that used to be rare or require vast and expensive laboratories are becoming simple and turn key, as has been the case with X-rays and urinalysis, and are broadening the scope of primary care. At Atrinea, we expect and are readying ourselves to employ these technologies as soon as insurance companies decide to support.

Treadmill stress tests have been a cheap, but imprecise diagnostic test for coronary artery disease. To be accurate a treadmill test would require that a patient had developed severe CAD requiring a minimum of 80% stenosis of the coronary arteries. CT scans have become the new standard for diagnosis. With a routine 64 slice CT, the arteries can be enlarged to the size of computer monitor, allowing radiologists to see any minor aberrations or abnormalities in the heart. CT scans are still extremely expensive, and primary care facilities do not have the patient volume to support one, but I believe this price point to be somewhat artificial and supported by the payment system for the tests. Atrinea is prepared for a wave of new cheap CT solutions for these simple exams and sees them as a routine, in office test that will yield dramatic cost savings and preventive benefits to patients and payers soon.

A technological industry that is already gaining ground, but does not have the financial incentive to take over yet is in comprehensive, black box blood testing machines. Simple machines have always existed for glucose, A1C, and hemoglobin tests, but already complete full metabolic panels, cholesterol testing, STD, PSA and thyroid tests, but payers continue to support large scale labs for doctors to send their patients to. Soon, I believe that payers will recognize that having these tests immediately available in a self-contained, in-practice machine will warrant payment directly to physicians. Saving payers substantial fees in testing and office visits(often sharing all normal results).

The phenomenon of seeing patients routinely with normal test results is another forced upon physicians by payers. Our and many providers are ready to complete simple over the phone visits as soon as payers recognize the provider time required and pay for their services.

One final technology that is quickly becoming affordable and is continuing to show tremendous preventive potential is in DNA sequencing. With DNA, a whole new world of precise care is developing known as personal medicine. Unlike CT angiograms and blood tests, DNA sequencing will never have to be repeated and as knowledge broadens, patients will learn more and more about their personal medical needs. Drug-gene interactions, risk profiling and mutational diseases are all simple given a patients DNA sequence. In 2001, the cost of sequencing an entire genome was about $100,000,000. It followed a fairly linear downward trend, costing little 10 million in late 2007. Prices then took an extremely sharp turn and were about $10000 at the end of 2011.

Sites like *www.23andMe.com* have found an affordable solution by taking 500,000 or so SNPs, or snips, instead of an entire DNA sequence for prices starting at $5000 and now about $200 dollars. These snips are valuable, but incomplete information and will likely be consumed by cheaper whole-genome sequencing. IBM recently sent out a press release documenting their progress with a machine that could likely sequence an entire genome for near $100. The precision of DNA based personal medicine allows it to be a perfect technology and set of services for primary care facilities to adopt.

The general trend of precision medical technology moving from expensive boutique or theoretical testing into affordable deliverable care has been constant. The testing equipment remains expensive and dangerous enough that doctors' and trained technicians are still required at the point of service. This is a perfect market for primary physicians to reach into, and creates a reality that insurers will not long be able to ignore.

Part III: Looking Forward

Glossary

AAFP—American Academy of Family Physicians—Founded in 1947 as the American Academy of General Practice, the AAFP changed its name to fit with Family Practice being formalized as the 20th American specialty in 1969. With over 100,000 members, the AAFP continues to focus on its founding objectives: advocacy, practice enhancement, education and health of the public.

ABFM—American board of Family Medicine—Founded in 1969 as the American board of family practice, the ABFM is the second largest certifying specialty board in the United States. Focused on certifying physicians and ensure continuing medical education for its members, the ABFM aims to ensure clinical excellence amongst all family practitioners.

ACO—Accountable Care Organization—With the advent of the medical home, ACO's emerged as a model for physicians to interact with payers in a way that moves away from the older volume based reimbursement systems and instead creates tiered metrics based on cost savings, quality metrics, and patient populations.

AMA—American Medical Association—Founded in 1847, the AMA is a professional organization with over 200,000 Physician members aimed at promoting public health through the refinement of medical practice.

APSSO—Assessment-Plan-Systems-Subjective-Objective—Our rearrangement of the SOAP acronym in a way that focusses on the readers of the information instead of the writers.

CMS—Center for Medicare & Medicaid Services—The administrator of the National Medicare and Medicaid programs.

EMR—Electronic Medical Record—A computerized version of a physicians medical records.

FFM—Future of Family Medicine—A project inaugurated by leading Family practice organizations from 7 countries in 2002. Assembled in response to the looming environment for primary care, the FFM project first outlined the idea of a Patient Centered Medical Home in their 2004 report.

HIPAA—Health Insurance Portability and Accountability Act of 1996—A national law passed with the emergence of new information technologies in order to protect patient privacy and set standards for electronic health information.

HIT—Health Information Technology—All of the computer systems required in running a health care practice. Including but not limited to: EMR, PHR, Patient Tracking, Registries, Lab interfaces, and billing software.

HMO--Health maintenance organization—Established in 1973, a healthcare benefit model that worked with managed care organizations on prepaid contracts.

IPA—Independent Practice Association—An association between individual physicians for negotiating with and contracting with payers as a group.

MA—Medical Assistant—A supportive non-licensed clinical and professional employee key to a physician's smooth clinical operations.

MCO—Managed Care Organization—Any one of the many models through which a group of physicians and or hospitals can organize to provide care to payers and other customers in a more organized fashion.

MRS—Medical Records Specialist—A person charged with ensuring a provider's care-giving is properly documented for health management, fiscal accountability and quality care.

NCQA—National Committee for Quality Assurance—Although previously known for accrediting health plans primarily, the NCQA is the organization through which we choose to certify our Patient Centered Medical Homes.

NMAFP—New Mexico Academy of Family Physicians—New Mexico's specialty association for Family Practice.

PCMH –Patient Centered Medical Home—A Model for primary care delivery first outlined in the 2004 FFM report. The term itself was borrowed from Pediatric literature.

PCPCC—Patient-Centered Primary Care Collaborative—A coalition of organizations (ourselves one) to develop and advance the role of Primary care and the PCMH model to deliver better care.

PPACA—Patient Protection and Affordable Care Act—Commonly called Obamacare, the PPACA is a broad legislative act passed in the United States in 2010.

PHR—Personal Health Record—A Patient's own copy of their health information, emerging as a more and more important factor with the continued focus on preventive care and health maintenance in PCMHs.

RBRVS--Resource-Based Relative Value Scale—A method used to determine how much providers should be paid based of specialty, location and specific care given.

SFFHC—Santa Fe Family Health Center—Transitioning out of solo practice, SFFHC was my first expansion of hours and physicians into a retail area in Santa Fe.

SOAP—Subjective, Objective, Assessment, Plan—The traditional model for documenting office visits.

BIBLIOGRAPHY

LINKS:

WWW.PBRIGGSLINKS.COM
This is our always up-to-date website for links to all of our facilities websites as well as relevant news, videos, articles and anything else we at Atrinea find interesting.

 *HTTP://WWW.ANNFAMMED.ORG/CONTENT/2/SUPPL_1/S3.FULL.PDF*
This is a link to a PDF of the Future of Family Medicine Report published by The Future of Family Medicine Project Leadership Committee in 2004. One of the most important pieces written about primary care recently.

WWW.TED.COM/TALKS/DANIEL_KRAFT_MEDICINE_S_FUTURE.HTML
The best TED talk we've ever seen. Daniel Kraft speaks in Maastricht on the future of medical applications and the role innovation is having in Medicine's future. A great primer on what we are excitedly watching come to health.

 *HTTP://WWW.FORBES.COM/SITES/DAVECHASE/2012/09/27/SOLVING-HEALTHCARE-REQUIRES-PRIMARY-CARE-RENAISSANCE/*
This is a recently published article in Forbes reassuring our confidence in the future of family care. As an entrepreneur, Dave Chase notes the ideal environment that primary care finds itself in know for leveraging more from payers, more for doctors and a new economy to support primary care growth.

WWW.NCQA.ORG
The National Committee for quality assurance has long been the certifying body for private payers. Because of this, and the power we want to have working with payers as we move forward, their PCMH recognition was our choice to lead us as we built our model.

 *HTTP://DEMO.SFMEDICALGROUP.COM/VIEW/LOGIN.PHP*
This is a demo of APSSO, our emr solution discussed in Part three.
Login: Admin
Password: demo

www.ingramcontent.com/pod-product-compliance
Lightning Source LLC
Chambersburg PA
CBHW072335290526
45794CB00002B/890